BLACKWELL'S

UNDERGROUND CLINICAL VIGNETTES

INTERNAL MEDICINE, VOL. II, 2E

BLACKWELL'S
UNDERGROUND CLINICAL VIGNETTES

INTERNAL MEDICINE, VOL. II, 2E

VIKAS BHUSHAN, MD
University of California, San Francisco, Class of 1991
Series Editor, Diagnostic Radiologist

VISHAL PALL, MBBS
Government Medical College, Chandigarh, India, Class of 1996
Series Editor, U. of Texas, Galveston, Resident in Internal Medicine &
Preventive Medicine

TAO LE, MD
University of California, San Francisco, Class of 1996

ZUBIN DAMANIA, MD
University of California, San Francisco, Class of 1999

VIPAL SONI, MD
UCLA School of Medicine, Class of 1999

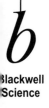

b

Blackwell
Science

CONTRIBUTORS

Charles Chiu, MD
University of California, San Francisco, Resident in Internal Medicine

Kalpita Shah, PA-C
University of Texas Medical Branch, Galveston, Class of 2000

Shalin Patel, MD
McGraw Medical Center, Northwestern University, Resident in Internal Medicine

Mae Sheikh-Ali, MD
University of Damascus, Syria, Class of 1999

Hoang Nguyen, MD, MBA
Northwestern University, Class of 2001

Sonal Shah, MD
Ross University, Class of 2000

FACULTY REVIEWER

Thomas A. Blackwell, MD
Program Director, Program in Internal Medicine
University of Texas Medical Branch, Galveston

© 2002 by Blackwell Science, Inc.

Editorial Offices:

Commerce Place, 350 Main Street, Malden,
    Massachusetts 02148, USA
Osney Mead, Oxford OX2 0EL, England
25 John Street, London WC1N 2BS, England
23 Ainslie Place, Edinburgh EH3 6AJ, Scotland
54 University Street, Carlton, Victoria 3053,
    Australia

Other Editorial Offices:

Blackwell Wissenschafts-Verlag GmbH,
    Kurfürstendamm 57, 10707 Berlin, Germany
Blackwell Science KK, MG Kodenmacho Building,
    7-10 Kodenmacho Nihombashi, Chuo-ku,
    Tokyo 104, Japan
Iowa State University Press, A Blackwell Science
    Company, 2121 S. State Avenue, Ames, Iowa
    50014-8300, USA

Distributors:

The Americas
Blackwell Publishing
c/o AIDC
P.O. Box 20
50 Winter Sport Lane
Williston, VT 05495-0020
(Telephone orders: 800-216-2522;
    fax orders: 802-864-7626)
Australia
Blackwell Science Pty, Ltd.
54 University Street
Carlton, Victoria 3053
(Telephone orders: 03-9347-0300;
    fax orders: 03-9349-3016)
Outside The Americas and Australia
Blackwell Science, Ltd.
c/o Marston Book Services, Ltd.
P.O. Box 269
Abingdon
Oxon OX14 4YN
England
(Telephone orders: 44-01235-465500;
    fax orders: 44-01235-465555)

Acquisitions: Laura DeYoung
Development: Amy Nuttbrock
Production: Lorna Hind and Shawn Girsberger
Manufacturing: Lisa Flanagan
Marketing Manager: Kathleen Mulcahy
Cover design by Leslie Haimes
Interior design by Shawn Girsberger
Typeset by TechBooks
Printed and bound by Capital City Press

Blackwell's Underground Clinical Vignettes:
    Internal Medicine II, 2e
ISBN 0-632-04565-5

Printed in the United States of America
02 03 04 05 5 4 3 2 1

The Blackwell Science logo is a trade mark of
Blackwell Science Ltd., registered at the United
Kingdom Trade Marks Registry

Library of Congress Cataloging-in-Publication Data
Bhushan, Vikas.
Blackwell's underground clinical vignettes.
Internal medicine / author, Vikas Bhushan. – 2nd ed.
    p. ; cm. – (Underground clinical vignettes) Rev. ed.
of: Internal medicine / Vikas Bhushan ... [et al.].
c1999. ISBN 0-632-04563-9 (pbk.)
1. Internal medicine – Case studies. 2. Physicians –
Licenses – United States – Examinations – Study
guides.
    [DNLM: 1. Internal Medicine – Case Report.
2. Internal Medicine – Problems and Exercises.
WB 18.2 B575ba 2002] I. Title: Underground
clinical vignettes. Internal medicine. II. Title:
Internal medicine. III. Title. IV. Series.
    RC66 .B48 2002
    616'.0076–dc21

                                    2001004893

CONTENTS

MINICASES

ACKNOWLEDGMENTS

Throughout the production of this book, we have had the support of many friends and colleagues. Special thanks to our support team including Anu Gupta, Andrea Fellows, Anastasia Anderson, Srishti Gupta, Mona Pall, Jonathan Kirsch and Chirag Amin. For prior contributions we thank Gianni Le Nguyen, Tarun Mathur, Alex Grimm, Sonia Santos and Elizabeth Sanders.

We have enjoyed working with a world-class international publishing group at Blackwell Science, including Laura DeYoung, Amy Nuttbrock, Lisa Flanagan, Shawn Girsberger, Lorna Hind and Gordon Tibbitts. For help with securing images for the entire series we also thank Lee Martin, Kristopher Jones, Tina Panizzi and Peter Anderson at the University of Alabama, the Armed Forces Institute of Pathology, and many of our fellow Blackwell Science authors.

For submitting comments, corrections, editing, proofreading, and assistance across all of the vignette titles in all editions, we collectively thank:

Tara Adamovich, Carolyn Alexander, Kris Alden, Henry E. Aryan, Lynman Bacolor, Natalie Barteneva, Dean Bartholomew, Debashish Behera, Sumit Bhatia, Sanjay Bindra, Dave Brinton, Julianne Brown, Alexander Brownie, Tamara Callahan, David Canes, Bryan Casey, Aaron Caughey, Hebert Chen, Jonathan Cheng, Arnold Cheung, Arnold Chin, Simion Chiosea, Yoon Cho, Samuel Chung, Gretchen Conant, Vladimir Coric, Christopher Cosgrove, Ronald Cowan, Karekin R. Cunningham, A. Sean Dalley, Rama Dandamudi, Sunit Das, Ryan Armando Dave, John David, Emmanuel de la Cruz, Robert DeMello, Navneet Dhillon, Sharmila Dissanaike, David Donson, Adolf Etchegaray, Alea Eusebio, Priscilla A. Frase, David Frenz, Kristin Gaumer, Yohannes Gebreegziabher, Anil Gehi, Tony George, L.M. Gotanco, Parul Goyal, Alex Grimm, Rajeev Gupta, Ahmad Halim, Sue Hall, David Hasselbacher, Tamra Heimert, Michelle Higley, Dan Hoit, Eric Jackson, Tim Jackson, Sundar Jayaraman, Pei-Ni Jone, Aarchan Joshi, Rajni K. Jutla, Faiyaz Kapadi, Seth Karp, Aaron S. Kesselheim, Sana Khan, Andrew Pin-wei Ko, Francis Kong, Paul Konitzky, Warren S. Krackov, Benjamin H.S. Lau, Ann LaCasce, Connie Lee, Scott Lee, Guillermo Lehmann, Kevin Leung, Paul Levett, Warren Levinson, Eric Ley, Ken Lin,

Pavel Lobanov, J. Mark Maddox, Aram Mardian, Samir Mehta, Gil Melmed, Joe Messina, Robert Mosca, Michael Murphy, Vivek Nandkarni, Siva Naraynan, Carvell Nguyen, Linh Nguyen, Deanna Nobleza, Craig Nodurft, George Noumi, Darin T. Okuda, Adam L. Palance, Paul Pamphrus, Jinha Park, Sonny Patel, Ricardo Pietrobon, Riva L. Rahl, Aashita Randeria, Rachan Reddy, Beatriu Reig, Marilou Reyes, Jeremy Richmon, Tai Roe, Rick Roller, Rajiv Roy, Diego Ruiz, Anthony Russell, Sanjay Sahgal, Urmimala Sarkar, John Schilling, Isabell Schmitt, Daren Schuhmacher, Sonal Shah, Edie Shen, Justin Smith, John Stulak, Lillian Su, Julie Sundaram, Rita Suri, Seth Sweetser, Antonio Talayero, Merita Tan, Mark Tanaka, Eric Taylor, Jess Thompson, Indi Trehan, Raymond Turner, Okafo Uchenna, Eric Uyguanco, Richa Varma, John Wages, Alan Wang, Eunice Wang, Andy Weiss, Amy Williams, Brian Yang, Hany Zaky, Ashraf Zaman and David Zipf.

For generously contributing images to the entire *Underground Clinical Vignette* Step 2 series, we collectively thank the staff at Blackwell Science in Oxford, Boston, and Berlin as well as:

- Alfred Cuschieri, Thomas P.J. Hennessy, Roger M. Greenhalgh, David I. Rowley, Pierce A. Grace (*Clinical Surgery*, © 1996 Blackwell Science), Figures 13.23, 13.35b, 13.51, 15.13, 15.2.

- John Axford (*Medicine*, © 1996 Blackwell Science), Figures f3.10, 2.103a, 2.110b, 3.20a, 3.20b, 3.25b, 3.38a, 5.9Bi, 5.9Bii, 6.41a, 6.41b, 6.74b, 6.74c, 7.78ai, 7.78aii, 7.78b, 8.47b, 9.9e, f3.17, f3.36, f3.37, f5.27, f5.28, f5.45a, f5.48, f5.49a, f5.50, f5.65a, f5.67, f5.68, f8.27a, 10.120b, 11.63b, 11.63c, 11.68a, 11.68b, 11.68c, 12.37a, 12.37b.

- Peter Armstrong, Martin L. Wastie (*Diagnostic Imaging, 4th Edition*, © 1998 Blackwell Science), Figures 2.100, 2.108d, 2.109, 2.11, 2.112, 2.121, 2.122, 2.13, 2.1ba, 2.1bb, 2.36, 2.53, 2.54, 2.69a, 2.71, 2.80a, 2.81b, 2.82, 2.84a, 2.84b, 2.88, 2.89a, 2.89b, 2.90b, 2.94a, 2.94b, 2.96, 2.97, 2.98a, 2.98c, 3.11, 3.19, 3.20, 3.21, 3.22, 3.28, 3.30, 3.34, 3.35b, 3.35c, 3.36, 4.7, 4.8, 4.9, 5.29, 5.33, 5.58, 5.62, 5.63, 5.64, 5.65b, 5.66a, 5.66b, 5.69, 5.71, 5.75, 5.8, 5.9, 6.17a, 6.17b, 6.25, 6.28, 6.29c, 6.30, 7.13, 7.17a, 7.45a, 7.45b, 7.46, 7.50, 7.52, 7.53a, 7.57a, 7.58, 8.7a, 8.7b, 8.7c, 8.86, 8.8a, 8.96, 8.9a, 9.17a, 9.17b, 10.13a, 10.13b, 10.14a, 10.14b, 10.14c, 10.17a, 10.17b, 11.16b, 11.17a, 11.17b, 11.19, 11.23, 11.24, 11.2b, 11.2d, 11.30a, 11.30b, 12.12, 12.15,

12.18, 12.19, 12.3, 12.4, 12.8a, 12.8b, 13.13a, 13.18, 13.18a, 13.20, 13.22a, 13.22b, 13.29, 14.14a, 14.5, 14.6a, 15.25b, 15.29b, 15.31, 15.37, 17.4.

- N.C. Hughes-Jones, S.N. Wickramasinghe (*Lecture Notes On: Haematology, 6th Edition,* © 1996 Blackwell Science), Figures 2.1b, 2.2a, 3.14, 3.8, 4.3, 5.2b, 5.5a, 5.8, 7.1, 7.2, 7.3, 7.5, 8.1, 10.5b, 10.6, 11.1, plate 29, plate 34, plate 44, plate 45, plate 48, plate 5, plate 42.

- Thomas Grumme, Wolfgang Kluge, Konrad Kretzschmar, Andreas Roesler (*Cerebral and Spinal Computed Tomography, 3rd Edition,* © 1998 Blackwell Science), Figures 16.2b, 16.3, 16.6a, 17.1a, 18-1c, 18-5, 41.3c, 41.3d, 44.3, 46.8, 47.7, 48.2, 48.6a, 53.5, 55.2a, 55.2c, 56.2b, 57.1, 61.3a, 61.3b, 63.1a, 64.3a, 65.3c, 66.3b, 67.6, 70.1a, 70.3, 81.2a, 81.4, 82.2, 82.3, 84.6.

- P.R. Patel (*Lecture Notes On: Radiology,* © 1998 Blackwell Science), Figures 2.15, 2.16, 2.25, 2.26, 2.30, 2.31, 2.33, 2.36, 3.11, 3.16, 3.19, 3.4, 3.7, 4.19, 4.20, 4.38, 4.44, 4.45, 4.46, 4.47, 4.49, 4.5, 5.14, 5.6, 6.18, 6.19, 6.20, 6.21, 6.22, 6.31a, 6.31b, 7.18, 7.19, 7.21, 7.22, 7.32, 7.34, 7.41, 7.46a, 7.46b, 7.48, 7.49, 7.9, 8.2, 8.3, 8.4, 8.5, 8.8, 8.9, 9.12, 9.2, 9.3, 9.8, 9.9, 10.11, 10.16, 10.5.

- Ramsay Vallance (*An Atlas of Diagnostic Radiology in Gastroenterology,* © 1999 Blackwell Science), Figures 1.22, 2.57, 2.27, 2.55a, 2.58, 2.59, 2.63, 2.64, 2.65, 3.11, 3.3, 3.37, 3.39, 3.4, 4.6a, 4.8, 4.9, 5.1, 5.29, 5.63, 5.64b, 5.65b, 5.66b, 5.68a, 5.68b, 6.110, 6.15, 6.17, 6.23, 6.29b, 6.30, 6.39, 6.64a, 6.64b, 6.75, 6.78, 6.80, 7.57a, 7.57c, 7.60a, 8.17, 8.48, 8.53, 8.66, 9.11a, 9.15, 9.17, 9.23, 9.24, 9.25, 9.28, 9.30, 9.32a, 9.33, 9.43, 9.45, 9.55b, 9.57, 9.63, 9.64a, 9.64b, 9.64c, 9.66, 10.28, 10.36, 10.44, 10.6.

Please let us know if your name has been missed or misspelled and we will be happy to make the update in the next edition.

PREFACE TO THE 2ND EDITION

We were very pleased with the overwhelmingly positive student feedback for the 1st edition of our *Underground Clinical Vignettes* series. Well over 100,000 copies of the UCV books are in print and have been used by students all over the world.

Over the last two years we have accumulated and incorporated **over a thousand "updates"** and improvements suggested by you, our readers, including:

- many additions of specific boards and wards testable content
- deletions of redundant and overlapping cases
- reordering and reorganization of all cases in both series
- a new master index by case name in each Atlas
- correction of a few factual errors
- diagnosis and treatment updates
- addition of 5–20 new cases in every book
- and the addition of clinical exam photographs within *UCV— Anatomy*

And most important of all, the second edition sets now include two brand new **COLOR ATLAS** supplements, one for each Clinical Vignette series.

- The *UCV–Basic Science Color Atlas* (*Step 1*) includes over 250 color plates, divided into gross pathology, microscopic pathology (histology), hematology, and microbiology (smears).
- The *UCV–Clinical Science Color Atlas* (*Step 2*) has over 125 color plates, including patient images, dermatology, and funduscopy.

Each atlas image is descriptively captioned and linked to its corresponding Step 1 case, Step 2 case, and/or Step 2 MiniCase.

How Atlas Links Work:

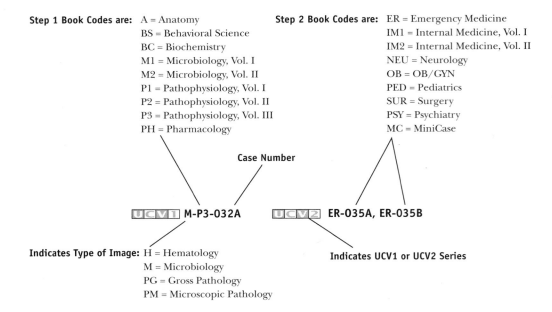

Step 1 Book Codes are:
A = Anatomy
BS = Behavioral Science
BC = Biochemistry
M1 = Microbiology, Vol. I
M2 = Microbiology, Vol. II
P1 = Pathophysiology, Vol. I
P2 = Pathophysiology, Vol. II
P3 = Pathophysiology, Vol. III
PH = Pharmacology

Step 2 Book Codes are:
ER = Emergency Medicine
IM1 = Internal Medicine, Vol. I
IM2 = Internal Medicine, Vol. II
NEU = Neurology
OB = OB/GYN
PED = Pediatrics
SUR = Surgery
PSY = Psychiatry
MC = MiniCase

Case Number

UCV1 M-P3-032A   UCV2 ER-035A, ER-035B

Indicates Type of Image:
H = Hematology
M = Microbiology
PG = Gross Pathology
PM = Microscopic Pathology

Indicates UCV1 or UCV2 Series

- If the Case number (032, 035, etc.) is not followed by a letter, then there is only one image. Otherwise A, B, C, D indicate up to 4 images.

Bold Faced Links: In order to give you access to the largest number of images possible, we have chosen to cross link the Step 1 and 2 series.

- If the link is bold-faced this indicates that the link is direct (i.e., Step 1 Case with the Basic Science Step 1 Atlas link).

- If the link is not bold-faced this indicates that the link is indirect (Step 1 case with Clinical Science Step 2 Atlas link or vice versa).

We have also implemented a few structural changes upon your request:

- Each current and future edition of our popular *First Aid for the USMLE Step 1* (Appleton & Lange/McGraw-Hill) and *First Aid for the USMLE Step 2* (Appleton & Lange/McGraw-Hill) book will be linked to the corresponding UCV case.

- We eliminated UCV → First Aid links as they frequently become out of date, as the *First Aid* books are revised yearly.

- The Color Atlas is also specially designed for quizzing—captions are descriptive and do not give away the case name directly.

New "MiniCases" replace the previous "Associated Diseases." There are now over **350 unique MiniCases** distributed throughout the *Step 2 Clinical* series, selected based on recent USMLE recollections.

We hope the updated UCV series will remain a unique and well-integrated study tool that provides compact clinical correlations to basic science information. They are designed to be easy and fun (comparatively) to read, and helpful for both licensing exams and the wards.

We invite your corrections and suggestions for the fourth edition of these books. For the first submission of each factual correction or new vignette that is selected for inclusion in the fourth edition, you will receive a personal acknowledgment in the revised book. If you submit over 20 high-quality corrections, additions or new vignettes we will also consider **inviting you to become a "Contributor" on the book of your choice**. If you are interested in becoming a potential "Contributor" or "Author" on a future UCV book, or working with our team in developing additional books, please also e-mail us your CV/resume.

We prefer that you submit corrections or suggestions via electronic mail to **UCVteam@yahoo.com**. Please include "Underground Vignettes" as the subject of your message. If you do not have access to e-mail, use the following mailing address: Blackwell Publishing, Attn: UCV Editors, 350 Main Street, Malden, MA 02148, USA.

Vikas Bhushan
Vishal Pall
Tao Le
October 2001

HOW TO USE THIS BOOK

This series was originally developed to address the increasing number of clinical vignette questions on medical examinations, including the USMLE Step 1 and Step 2. It is also designed to supplement and complement the popular *First Aid for the USMLE Step 1* (Appleton & Lange/McGraw Hill) and *First Aid for the USMLE Step 2* (Appleton & Lange/McGraw Hill).

Each UCV 2 book uses a series of approximately 50 **"supra-prototypical" cases as a way to condense testable facts and associations**. The clinical vignettes in this series are designed to give added emphasis to pathogenesis, epidemiology, management and complications. They also contain relevant extensive B/W imaging plates within each book. Additionally, each UCV2 book contains approximately 30 to 60 "MiniCases" that focus on presenting only the key facts for that disease in a tightly edited fashion.

Although each case tends to present all the signs, symptoms, and diagnostic findings for a particular illness, **patients generally will not present with such a "complete" picture either clinically or on a medical examination**. Cases are not meant to simulate a potential real patient or an exam vignette. All the **boldfaced "buzzwords" are for learning purposes** and are not necessarily expected to be found in any one patient with the disease.

Definitions of selected important terms are placed within the vignettes in (SMALL CAPS) in parentheses. Other parenthetical remarks often refer to the pathophysiology or mechanism of disease. The format should also help students learn to present cases succinctly during oral "bullet" presentations on clinical rotations. The cases are meant to serve as a condensed review, not as a primary reference. The information provided in this book has been prepared with a great deal of thought and careful research. This book should not, however, be considered as your sole source of information. Corrections, suggestions and submissions of new cases are encouraged and will be acknowledged and incorporated when appropriate in future editions.

ABBREVIATIONS

5-ASA	5-aminosalicylic acid
ABGs	arterial blood gases
ABVD	adriamycin/bleomycin/vincristine/dacarbazine
ACE	angiotensin-converting enzyme
ACTH	adrenocorticotropic hormone
ADH	antidiuretic hormone
AFP	alpha fetal protein
AI	aortic insufficiency
AIDS	acquired immunodeficiency syndrome
ALL	acute lymphocytic leukemia
ALT	alanine transaminase
AML	acute myelogenous leukemia
ANA	antinuclear antibody
ARDS	adult respiratory distress syndrome
ASD	atrial septal defect
ASO	anti-streptolysin O
AST	aspartate transaminase
AV	arteriovenous
BE	barium enema
BP	blood pressure
BUN	blood urea nitrogen
CAD	coronary artery disease
CALLA	common acute lymphoblastic leukemia antigen
CBC	complete blood count
CHF	congestive heart failure
CK	creatine kinase
CLL	chronic lymphocytic leukemia
CML	chronic myelogenous leukemia
CMV	cytomegalovirus
CNS	central nervous system
COPD	chronic obstructive pulmonary disease
CPK	creatine phosphokinase
CSF	cerebrospinal fluid
CT	computed tomography
CVA	cerebrovascular accident
CXR	chest x-ray
DIC	disseminated intravascular coagulation
DIP	distal interphalangeal
DKA	diabetic ketoacidosis
DM	diabetes mellitus
DTRs	deep tendon reflexes
DVT	deep venous thrombosis

EBV	Epstein–Barr virus
ECG	electrocardiography
Echo	echocardiography
EF	ejection fraction
EGD	esophagogastroduodenoscopy
EMG	electromyography
ERCP	endoscopic retrograde cholangiopancreatography
ESR	erythrocyte sedimentation rate
FEV	forced expiratory volume
FNA	fine needle aspiration
FTA-ABS	fluorescent treponemal antibody absorption
FVC	forced vital capacity
GFR	glomerular filtration rate
GH	growth hormone
GI	gastrointestinal
GM-CSF	granulocyte macrophage colony stimulating factor
GU	genitourinary
HAV	hepatitis A virus
hcG	human chorionic gonadotrophin
HEENT	head, eyes, ears, nose, and throat
HIV	human immunodeficiency virus
HLA	human leukocyte antigen
HPI	history of present illness
HR	heart rate
HRIG	human rabies immune globulin
HS	hereditary spherocytosis
ID/CC	identification and chief complaint
IDDM	insulin-dependent diabetes mellitus
Ig	immunoglobulin
IGF	insulin-like growth factor
IM	intramuscular
JVP	jugular venous pressure
KUB	kidneys/ureter/bladder
LDH	lactate dehydrogenase
LES	lower esophageal sphincter
LFTs	liver function tests
LP	lumbar puncture
LV	left ventricular
LVH	left ventricular hypertrophy
Lytes	electrolytes
MCHC	mean corpuscular hemoglobin concentration
MCV	mean corpuscular volume
MEN	multiple endocrine neoplasia

MGUS	monoclonal gammopathy of undetermined significance
MHC	major histocompatibility complex
MI	myocardial infarction
MOPP	mechlorethamine/vincristine (Oncovorin)/procarbazine/prednisone
MR	magnetic resonance (imaging)
NHL	non-Hodgkin's lymphoma
NIDDM	non-insulin-dependent diabetes mellitus
NPO	nil per os (nothing by mouth)
NSAID	nonsteroidal anti-inflammatory drug
PA	posteroanterior
PIP	proximal interphalangeal
PBS	peripheral blood smear
PE	physical exam
PFTs	pulmonary function tests
PMI	point of maximal intensity
PMN	polymorphonuclear leukocyte
PT	prothrombin time
PTCA	percutaneous transluminal angioplasty
PTH	parathyroid hormone
PTT	partial thromboplastin time
PUD	peptic ulcer disease
RBC	red blood cell
RPR	rapid plasma reagin
RR	respiratory rate
RS	Reed–Sternberg (cell)
RV	right ventricular
RVH	right ventricular hypertrophy
SBFT	small bowel follow-through
SIADH	syndrome of inappropriate secretion of ADH
SLE	systemic lupus erythematosus
STD	sexually transmitted disease
TFTs	thyroid function tests
tPA	tissue plasminogen activator
TSH	thyroid-stimulating hormone
TIBC	total iron-binding capacity
TIPS	transjugular intrahepatic portosystemic shunt
TPO	thyroid peroxidase
TSH	thyroid-stimulating hormone
TTP	thrombotic thrombocytopenic purpura
UA	urinalysis
UGI	upper GI
US	ultrasound

VDRL	Venereal Disease Research Laboratory
VS	vital signs
VT	ventricular tachycardia
WBC	white blood cell
WPW	Wolff–Parkinson–White (syndrome)
XR	x-ray

ID/CC A 25-year-old **male** with a history of **IV drug abuse** presents to the ER complaining of **high fever with chills** and weakness.

HPI Over the past 2 weeks, the patient has had **intermittent spiking fevers** with **night sweats** and chills as well as associated **joint pain** (ARTHRALGIA). Recently, he has also become confused and disoriented.

PE VS: **fever** (39.5°C); tachycardia (HR 118); tachypnea (RR 25); normal BP. PE: pallor; 3/6 holosystolic **murmur** increasing with inspiration; tender, pulsatile liver edge; **Roth's spots** observed on funduscopy; **Janeway lesions, Osler's nodules**, and petechiae on extremities.

Labs CBC: normocytic anemia; **leukocytosis** (16,300) with **left shift**. ESR and C-reactive protein elevated; **blood culture yields *Staphylococcus aureus*.**

Imaging Echo (transesophageal): large **vegetations on the tricuspid valve; tricuspid regurgitation**.

Pathogenesis Infectious endocarditis (IE) is characterized by the presence of valvular vegetations (composed of platelets and fibrin seeded by microorganisms carried in the blood) that tend to occur in areas of turbulent blood flow. While organisms that are generally minimally pathogenic, such as viridans streptococci, rely on prior endocardial insults (subacute IE), aggressive organisms such as *S. aureus* may infect normal valves (acute IE).

Epidemiology Endocarditis in native valves **occurs more frequently in men** and affects patients of all ages. However, 60% to 80% of patients have an underlying cardiac lesion (rheumatic heart disease, congenital heart lesions, mitral valve prolapse, aortic stenosis, or a prosthetic valve) that predisposes them to endocarditis. The most commonly involved valves are, in order of frequency, the **mitral, aortic, tricuspid, and pulmonary valves**. Streptococci are the predominant organism in native valves of non–IV drug abusers. Among **IV drug abusers** (commonly young males), the **tricuspid valve** is most commonly involved and *S. aureus* is the most common pathogen.

Management **IV antibiotics for 2 to 6 weeks** directed at the causative organism. **Empiric therapy is directed against gram-positive organisms. Valve replacement** is necessary in fungal or pseudomonal endocarditis, refractory CHF (due to valve incompetence), recurrent emboli, persistent bacteremia, complicated prosthetic valve involvement, and major myocardial involvement. After discharge, patients require lifelong **antibiotic prophylaxis** (amoxicillin or erythromycin) prior to dental work and other invasive procedures. Anticoagulation is not recommended.

Complications **Valvular destruction** may lead to pulmonary edema and CHF. **Septic emboli** may also occur, leading to distant infarction or infections. Deposition of immune complexes in the kidney may lead to **glomerulonephritis**. Local spread of infection may cause myocardial abscess, aortic root abscess, pericarditis, and myocardial infarction.

Atlas Link UCV1 PG-M1-001

ID/CC   A 40-year-old female complains of **fever**, loss of appetite, and disabling **weakness** of 2 months' duration.

HPI   She has been diagnosed with **rheumatic heart disease**, for which she has been receiving penicillin prophylaxis. She underwent a tooth extraction a month ago but did not take the prescribed prophylactic antibiotics. For the past 2 days, she has also had **hematuria** and a **skin rash**.

PE   VS: fever; tachycardia. PE: ill-appearing; pallor; petechial rash over body; small, tender nodules on finger pads (OSLER'S NODES); tiny hemorrhages on palms and soles (JANEWAY LESIONS); clubbing of fingers; subungual **splinter hemorrhages** and conjunctival hemorrhage; oval white spots in retina (ROTH'S SPOTS); JVP normal; **splenomegaly**; "rumbling" mid-diastolic **murmur** with presystolic accentuation at apex; opening snap at apex (suggestive of **mitral stenosis**).

Labs   CBC: anemia; leukocytosis. Elevated ESR. UA: proteinuria; hematuria; RBC casts. Three blood cultures taken 2 hours apart yield **viridans group streptococcus**.

Imaging   CXR, PA: superior displacement of the left main bronchus; double atrial shadow; straightening of the left heart border and pulmonary venous congestion. Echo (with doppler): mitral valve vegetations.

Pathogenesis   Acute endocarditis involves normal heart valves, is rapidly progressive, and is often fatal in < 6 weeks. **Subacute bacterial endocarditis** (SBE) is more **chronic (> 6 weeks)** and involves bacteria of relatively low virulence that are part of the normal flora. These agents are not sufficiently invasive to initiate infection in normal heart valves but may do so on **damaged or congenitally deformed valves**. More than 50% of SBE cases are caused by streptococcal species; the most common organism is *Streptococcus viridans*, which is commonly found on the **oral mucosa**. Release into the bloodstream can occur with oral manipulation; hence the need for prophylactic antibiotics prior to dental procedures. In contrast, the portal of entry for *Streptococcus bovis* usually arises from malignant or premalignant colonic lesions. **Enterococcal endocarditis** usually results from instrumentation or trauma to the lower GI or GU tract in the elderly (colonized with *Enterococcus faecalis*).

Epidemiology   Native valve endocarditis affects **males more often than females**, and most patients are older than 50; the majority have a

predisposing cardiac lesion. Rheumatic valvular disease accounts for some 30% of cases. The mitral valve is most commonly involved, followed by the aortic valve; right-sided endocarditis is rare. Congenital heart disease other than valve prolapse (PDA, VSD, tetralogy of Fallot, coarctation of the aorta, pulmonary stenosis, and bicuspid aortic valve) is the underlying lesion in 10% to 20% of cases of endocarditis. **Degenerative valve disease** (calcific aortic stenosis in the elderly) also predisposes to infective endocarditis. No underlying heart disease is found in 20% to 40% of cases of infective endocarditis.

Management High-dose **parenteral antibiotics** for 4 to 6 weeks. **Viridans streptococci** constitute the most common pathogen in SBE; **penicillin** or **penicillin plus gentamicin** is the therapy of choice. If the patient has a **prosthetic valve**, suspect methicillin-resistant *S. epidermidis*; treat with **vancomycin, rifampin**, and **gentamicin**. In **IV drug abusers**, suspect *Staphylococcus aureus*; treat with **nafcillin** plus **gentamicin** or with vancomycin if blood cultures grow methicillin-resistant *S. aureus* (MRSA). Draw blood cultures periodically; cultures typically become negative within a few days following the initiation of antibiotic therapy. Surgery may be necessary for refractory endocarditis, acute hemodynamic abnormalities, or recurrent embolizations. Patients with valvular disease or prosthetic heart valves should receive **antibiotic prophylaxis** prior to dental or surgical procedures.

Complications Acute valvular regurgitation, pulmonary edema, and heart failure may result from valve destruction. Local spread of infection may lead to pericarditis and to aortic root or myocardial abscesses. Septic emboli may result in brain abscess or cerebritis.

Atlas Link ⓊⒸⓋ❶ PG-M1-005

ID/CC   A **68-year-old white male** who works as a **farmer** complains of several discrete dry, rough, scaly lesions on his **forehead**.

HPI   He has worked **outdoors** for many years and has **never used sunscreen**. He states that he first noticed the lesions several months ago but adds that they are not painful unless he runs his fingers over them.

PE   VS: normal. PE: **fair-skinned** with **blond hair** and **blue eyes**; numerous small (< 1 cm), coarse, yellow-brown lesions with reddish tinge on forehead, ears, posterior neck, and dorsal aspect of hands (sun-exposed regions).

Labs   Skin biopsy shows **epidermal pleomorphic keratinocytes**.

Pathogenesis   Actinic or solar keratosis results from repeated and prolonged exposure to ultraviolet light (primarily UVB 290 to 320 nm), ionizing radiation, or polycyclic aromatic hydrocarbons and arsenicals, leading to damage to keratinocytes. Clonal expansion of mutated forms of the tumor suppressor gene p53 has been observed in cases of both actinic keratosis and squamous cell carcinoma, indicating that actinic keratosis is indeed a **premalignant lesion** that may be regarded as **squamous cell carcinoma in situ**.

Epidemiology   Actinic keratosis, like squamous cell carcinoma of the skin, occurs with increased frequency among **males**, individuals with a **light complexion**, those who **work outdoors**, people who frequent tanning salons, and individuals from Australia or the southwestern United States; the disease is rarely seen in blacks or East Indians. Immunosuppressed patients are also at increased risk.

Management   The initial treatment of uncomplicated lesions involves the **topical application of 5-FU and/or liquid nitrogen**. A **skin biopsy** may be necessary to rule out squamous cell carcinoma if evidence of ulceration or induration is present. Extensive skin involvement or evidence of nodular lesions requires **surgical excision**. Prevention primarily involves the use of **UVA/UVB sunscreens**.

Complications   Approximately 1 in 1,000 solar keratosis lesions will develop into invasive squamous cell carcinoma each year.

ACTINIC KERATOSIS

ID/CC	A 44-year-old male complains of **sore, scaly hands**.
HPI	The patient states that he has worked as a **bricklayer** (chronic exposure to chromate salts in cement) for the past 20 years. He adds that the condition of his hands has gradually worsened over the past year.
PE	VS: normal. PE: **bilateral hyperkeratosis, maceration, fissuring, and erosion of palms and proximal portion of each digit.**
Labs	**Patch test** elicits a local response at a distant site.
Pathogenesis	Contact dermatitis appears in two forms: **nonallergic** (caused by chemical irritation) and **allergic/eczematous (type IV hypersensitivity reaction to an antigen)**. Acids and bases cause irritant contact dermatitis, while poison ivy and oak usually cause allergic contact dermatitis. Irritant contact dermatitis is concentration dependent and sharply marginated and does not require sensitization (unlike allergic contact dermatitis, which depends on sensitization). Chronic toxic or irritant dermatitis results from repeated exposure to agents that gradually erode the barrier function of the skin and ultimately elicit an inflammatory response.
Epidemiology	Occupational exposures play a crucial role in the etiology of contact dermatitis. Young children only infrequently present with allergic contact dermatitis, and black individuals appear to be less susceptible.
Management	**Removal of offending agent; corticosteroids.** Additionally, one may drain large vesicles without uncovering them and apply wet dressings with Burow's solution every 3 hours for acute dermatitis.

CONTACT DERMATITIS

ID/CC	A 32-year-old man presents with an intensely **pruritic vesiculopapular** eruption limited to the extensor surfaces of his knees and elbows.
HPI	The patient reports **repeated episodes** of the rash over the past few years. The first episode occurred at age 24.
PE	VS: normal. PE: cardiopulmonary exam normal; pruritic vesiculopapular eruption on extensor surfaces of knees and elbows; remainder of exam normal.
Labs	Direct immunofluorescence of normal perilesional skin demonstrates granular deposits of IgA in papillary dermis and along epidermal basement membrane zone; no circulating IgA.
Pathogenesis	Dermatitis herpetiformis is an idiopathic autoimmune disease characterized by **granular deposits of IgA** in the papillary dermis and along the epidermal basement membrane zone with intensely pruritic, chronic vesiculopapular lesions symmetrically distributed over the extensor surfaces.
Epidemiology	Greater than 90% of patients with dermatitis herpetiformis are **HLA-B8/DRw3 and HLA-DQw2 positive**. Almost all have associated, usually subclinical **gluten-sensitive enteropathy**.
Management	Maintenance of a **gluten-free diet** may diminish outbreaks. **Dapsone** should be used in exacerbations.
Atlas Link	UCV2 IM2-005

MINICASE 131: ACNE VULGARIS

A common skin disorder caused by excess sebum production and follicular blockage/inflammation

- presents with comedones (follicular cysts) and inflammatory papules, pustules, or nodules, predominantly on the face and trunk
- treat with topical or oral antibiotics, topical keratolytics, or oral isotretinoin (teratogenic) for recalcitrant cases
- the condition usually resolves after adolescence

Atlas Link: UCV2 MC-131

DERMATITIS HERPETIFORMIS

ID/CC	A **23-year-old female** presents to the clinic complaining of **painful, tender nodules on the anterior surface of her leg**.
HPI	She had a **fever** and **sore throat** prior to the appearance of the lesions. She also complains of an **aching pain in her ankles**.
PE	VS: **fever** (38.6°C). PE: **numerous deep red** (ERYTHEMATOUS), round lesions 3 to 20 cm in diameter that are poorly demarcated and located on lower legs bilaterally; palpable nodules that are indurated and tender.
Labs	ESR elevated; throat culture positive for group A β-hemolytic streptococci (GABHS).
Imaging	CXR: normal.
Pathogenesis	Erythema nodosum is an acute inflammatory or immunologic disorder leading to a septal panniculitis in subcutaneous fat. It arises in **response to infectious agents** (e.g., GABHS, *Yersinia*, histoplasmosis, **coccidioidomycosis**, and tuberculosis), in **inflammatory conditions** such as sarcoidosis and **ulcerative colitis**, and in response to **drugs** such as sulfonamides and OCPs. Generally, the condition remits spontaneously within 6 weeks.
Epidemiology	The most common cause of acute panniculitis. Patients are generally **female** (3:1) and **between the ages of 15 and 30**.
Management	Treatment is generally symptomatic and includes bed rest, decreased weight bearing, compressive bandages, and/or NSAIDs. In severe cases where infectious agents have been ruled out, prednisone may be administered.
Complications	Complications are related to the underlying disease.
Atlas Link	UCV2 IM2-006

MINICASE 132: ATOPIC DERMATITIS

An idiopathic, chronic, IgE-mediated skin inflammation
- presents with intense pruritus, lichenification secondary to scratching, erythema, and scaling
- treat with topical corticosteroids, hydrating creams, and removal of potential allergens
- complications include secondary infection

ID/CC A 34-year-old **homosexual** male presents with unusual **purple-red, painless skin lesions** about the face and neck.

HPI He also complains of shortness of breath and adds that he has had dull chest pain and a limited appetite and has **coughed up blood** on a few occasions (HEMOPTYSIS). He has been **HIV positive** for 6 years.

PE VS: normal. PE: pallor; multiple mucocutaneous **purplish macules**; palpable abdominal masses and tenderness; generalized indurated lymphadenopathy; pedal edema.

Labs CBC: anemia; thrombocytosis; lymphopenia. **CD4 lymphocyte count decreased** (155×10^6/L); biopsy of lesion reveals **proliferation of spindle cells, endothelial cells**, and extravasation of RBCs.

Imaging CXR: bilateral lower lobe infiltrates obscure the margins of the mediastinum and diaphragm (finding suggestive of **pulmonary metastases**). Fiberoptic bronchoscopy and endoscopy for visualization and biopsy of other suspected Kaposi's sarcoma (KS) sites should be performed. Stage the tumor with a chest CT and bone scan.

Pathogenesis KS is a **hemangiosarcoma** that may affect the skin, viscera, and mucous membranes. The lymph nodes, GI tract, and lungs are also commonly involved. KS is usually seen as an "opportunistic" neoplasm in HIV-positive homosexual men but may be seen during any stage of the infection. Etiologic associations include Kaposi's sarcoma-associated virus (HHV-8).

Epidemiology KS in a male younger than 60 years is strongly suggestive of HIV infection. Ninety-six percent of AIDS-related cases occur in homosexual men. KS is rare in children and hemophiliacs with AIDS.

Management **Quiescent lesions require no specific therapy. Surgery** for cutaneous lesions and **resection of isolated lung metastases**. Few AIDS patients with KS die as a result of this malignancy; thus, treatment regimens that suppress the immune system should be avoided. Treatment may be indicated for lesions that are associated with significant discomfort (e.g., those located over a joint), dysphagia (e.g., oropharyngeal lesions), or cosmetic problems (e.g., facial lesions). **Interferon** is useful in early disease. **Combination chemotherapy** with doxorubicin, etoposide,

KAPOSI'S SARCOMA

vinblastine, and bleomycin is warranted in aggressive KS.
Prognosis is related to CD4 count and immune status.

Complications   Ulceration of the cutaneous lesion with subsequent infection is
a common side effect of therapy; GI obstruction and hemor-
rhage may occur with internal lesions.

Atlas Link   UCV2 IM2-007

MINICASE 133: CELLULITIS

A diffuse, acute spreading infection of the skin involving deeper tissues
- often caused by *Staphylococcus* or *Streptococcus* spp
- presents with pain, redness, swelling, and induration
- treat with cephalexin or dicloxacillin

MINICASE 134: DISCOID LUPUS ERYTHEMATOSUS

Dermal lupus associated with exposure to solar or UV radiation
- presents with localized erythematous plaques with thick adherent scales,
  predominantly on the face, scalp, and external ears, along with central scaling,
  atrophy, and depigmentation
- can cause scarring alopecia
- treat with topical corticosteroids, chloroquine, avoidance of sunlight

Atlas Link: UCV2 MC-134

MINICASE 135: DYSPLASTIC NEVI

Autosomal-dominant predisposition to develop nevi
- presents with multiple irregular-bordered nevi of pink, tan, and brown shades
- treat with excision if possible and sun protection
- nevi may develop into malignant melanoma

Atlas Link: UCV2 MC-135

MINICASE 136: ERYSIPELAS

Infection, commonly on the face, by *Streptococcus pyogenes*
- presents with characteristic bright red, raised macule with well-demarcated borders,
  fever, and pain
- treat with penicillin

Atlas Link: UCV2 MC-136

ID/CC	An 18-year-old man presents with **scaly salmon-pink lesions** on the extensor surfaces of his elbows and knees.
HPI	The patient is otherwise healthy.
PE	VS: normal. PE: **erythematous papules and plaques** with silver scaling on extensor surfaces of elbows and knees; nail pitting of hands.
Labs	Skin biopsy shows focal parakeratosis, hyperkeratosis, elongation and thickening of rete ridges, and thinning of epidermis above dermal papillae.
Pathogenesis	Psoriasis is an idiopathic disease, perhaps autoimmune in origin, that is characterized by epidermal proliferation with **increased thickness of the stratum spinosum** (ACANTHOSIS), **retention of nuclei in the cells of the stratum corneum** (PARAKERATOSIS) and collections of neutrophils (MONRO'S MICROABSCESSES) within the stratum corneum; it most often involves the **extensor surfaces** of the elbows and knees, scalp, and sacral areas.
Epidemiology	A common dermatologic disease. Thirty-five percent of patients have a family history of psoriasis.
Management	Mild to moderate psoriasis can be treated with **topical corticosteroids. Keratolytic agents** (e.g., salicylic acid) can be used when marked hyperkeratosis is present. **Tar compounds** may be beneficial when alternated with corticosteroids. Severe psoriasis should be treated **chemotherapeutically** (methotrexate, cyclosporin) and with **UV light**.
Complications	Extensive disease can lead to **psoriatic arthritis**. Secondary bacterial infection may occur as well (pustular psoriasis).
Atlas Links	UCV2 IM2-008A, IM2-008B, IM2-008C

MINICASE 137: ERYSIPELOID

Skin infection caused by *Erysipelothrix rhusiopathiae*, often acquired through contact with fish or swine
- presents with a well-demarcated reddish-purple plaque with severe pain, edema, and induration, usually involving the hand
- isolation of the organism from biopsy or blood is diagnostic
- treat with oral antibiotics (penicillin V, ciprofloxacin)
- rarely complicated by endocarditis

ID/CC	A 74-year-old man with Parkinson's disease presents with a greasy, **scaly rash** that has spread from his scalp to his eyebrows, eyelids, and nasolabial folds.
HPI	The patient reports increased itching over the involved areas. He had been treated for severe dandruff in the past year.
PE	VS: normal. PE: bilateral, symmetrically distributed patches of greasy, erythematous scales localized to hair-covered areas of the head and nasolabial folds.
Pathogenesis	Seborrheic dermatitis is a common, chronic disorder characterized by **greasy scales** overlying erythematous plaques or patches. Lesions are most commonly located on the scalp (may be recognized as severe dandruff) but may also affect the eyebrows, eyelids, glabella, nasolabial folds, or ears. Although the condition is more frequently seen in patients with Parkinson's disease, cerebrovascular accident, or HIV, the majority of individuals with seborrheic dermatitis have no underlying disorder. Its etiology is thought to be an inflammatory reaction to the yeast *Pityrosporum*.
Epidemiology	May be evident in the first weeks of life, commonly affecting the scalp (CRADLE CAP). It is rarely seen in children after infancy but is evident again in adulthood. Affects approximately 3% of the general population.
Management	Treat the scalp with 2.5% selenium sulfide, tar, salicylic acid, or ketoconazole shampoo. Apply **low-dose corticosteroids** or **ketoconazole** cream to the affected skin in severe cases.

ID/CC A **63-year-old white male** presents with a **reddish nodule** on the left side of his lip that has failed to heal for several months.

HPI The patient reports a **tendency to sunburn** due to his fair skin. He had another lesion in the same location that was diagnosed as **actinic keratosis** almost 10 years ago. The present lesion is not painful or pruritic.

PE VS: normal. PE: blond and **fair-skinned**; no acute distress; HEENT remarkable for 6.0- × 8.0-mm **red, conical, hard nodule with ulceration** on superior aspect of lower left lip margin.

Labs **Biopsy** of lesion reveals invasion of dermis by sheets and islands of neoplastic epidermal cells, often with **"keratin pearls."**

Pathogenesis Squamous cell carcinoma (SCC) is a malignant neoplasm of keratinizing epithelial cells. It may develop anywhere on the body but typically involves sun-damaged skin. Several premalignant forms should be noted, including actinic keratosis, actinic cheilitis, and Bowen's disease (may develop into SCC in 20% of cases).

Epidemiology Nonmelanoma skin cancer is the most common cancer in the United States, with > 800,000 cases diagnosed each year; SCC accounts for approximately 20% of cases (basal cell carcinoma accounts for 70% to 80%). The causes are multifactorial, including **cumulative exposure to UVB sunlight**, male sex, older age, Celtic ancestry, fair complexion, tendency to sunburn, and outdoor occupation.

Management **Surgical excision** is the mainstay of treatment; Mohs' microsurgery, radiation, and cryosurgery are alternate modalities. Metastases are treated with lymph node dissection, irradiation, or both. Because most cases are related to chronic UVB exposure, emphasis should be placed on prevention with regular use of **sunscreens** and protective clothing. Close follow-up for detection of recurrence, metastasis, or new cancers is indicated in all patients with a history of skin cancer.

Complications SCC carries a **low but significant malignant potential**. Metastases occur in 0.3% to 3.7% of patients with cutaneous lesions, 11% of ear lesions, and 13% of lower lip lesions; the rate of metastasis is higher for cancers arising in burn scars, chronic ulcerations, genitalia, and recurrent tumors. Regional lymph nodes are the most common site of metastasis. The prognosis is poor in patients with metastatic disease.

Atlas Links   UCV2   IM2-010A, IM-010B

MINICASE 138: ERYTHRODERMA

A systemic skin inflammation that is either idiopathic or secondary to underlying dermatologic disease (e.g., psoriasis, dermatitis), cutaneous lymphomas, or drug reactions
- presents with generalized pruritic erythema with lichenification and secondary scaling that may desquamate
- treat with corticosteroids and moisturizers
- treat the underlying condition if it can be determined
- complications include secondary infections, folate deficiency, hypoproteinemia, CHF, dehydration, and sepsis

---

MINICASE 139: FURUNCLE

A boil caused by *Staphylococcus aureus* infection of the hair follicle and subcutaneous tissue
- presents with pain, tenderness, and a fluctuant nodule
- treat with incision and drainage followed by penicillinase-resistant antibiotic therapy (e.g., nafcillin)
- risk factors for furunculosis (recurrent furuncles) are IV drug use, diabetes mellitus, and HIV

MINICASE 140: HUMAN PAPILLOMAVIRUS (HPV)—PLANTAR WARTS

Hyperkeratotic lesions on the plantar surface of the foot caused by infection with human papillomavirus (HPV) types 1, 2, or 4
- exposure is often associated with the use of public showers
- presents with foot and heel pain and with yellow-gray, hyperkeratotic lesions
- treat with topical keratolytic agents, cryotherapy, or surgery
- complications include secondary infection and transmission of virus

MINICASE 141: HUMAN PAPILLOMAVIRUS (HPV)—COMMON WART

Caused by infection with one of the more than 150 types of HPV
- may affect any area of the skin and mucous membranes and is estimated to occur in 7% to 12% of the world population
- common warts (verruca vulgaris) appear as hard papules with a rough, irregular surface
- diagnosis is usually clinical, but Southern blot hybridization for the HPV DNA is confirmatory
- may spontaneously regress, or treat with topical agents (salicylic acid, cantharidin, dinitrochlorobenzene, dibutyl squaric acid, trichloroacetic acid, or podophyllin), cryosurgery, or lasers

MINICASE 142: LICHEN PLANUS

An inflammatory, pruritic skin disease that is usually idiopathic
- presents with pruritic, violaceous, angulated 1- to 4-mm papules with fine white lines on the wrists, external genitalia, and oral and genital mucous membranes (distributed in a netlike pattern)
- treat with topical glucocorticoids with oral antihistamines for pruritus
- complications include a high rate of recurrence and rare neoplastic degeneration

Atlas Link: UCV2 MC-142

MINICASE 143: MOLLUSCUM CONTAGIOSUM

Viral infection of the skin acquired by skin-to-skin contact, often venereal
- common in AIDS patients
- presents with one or more dome-shaped, fleshy papules with central umbilications
- lesions are typically self-limiting
- may treat with cryotherapy

Atlas Link: UCV2 MC-143

MINICASE 144: MYCOSIS FUNGOIDES—SÉZARY SYNDROME

The leukemic phase of mycosis fungoides
- usually seen in middle-aged men
- presents with fever, malaise, and erythematous, scaly, extremely pruritic plaques
- Sézary cells seen on PBS
- treat with chemotherapy

Atlas Link: UCV2 MC-144

MINICASES: 141–144

MINICASE 145: OSLER–WEBER–RENDU DISEASE (HEREDITARY TELANGIECTASIA)

An autosomal-dominant genetic disorder with abnormal vascular proliferation causing telangiectatic skin lesions, pulmonary AV fistulas, and CNS vascular malformations
- presents with skin and mucosal telangiectases and GI or nasal bleeding
- lab findings include hypochromic microcytic anemia due to iron deficiency
- treat accessible lesions with pressure, styptics, or topical hemostatic agents, iron supplementation for iron deficiency anemia
- complications include brain abscess, ischemic stroke (paradoxical emboli), and severe bleeding episodes

Atlas Link: ⃞UⒸⓋ②⃞ MC-145

MINICASE 146: PEDICULOSIS

Ectoparasite infestation ("lice") spread by close contact or through fomites
- risk factors include overcrowding, sexual promiscuity, malnourishment, and poor hygiene
- presents with nocturnal itching
- examination reveals small erythematous papules on the back of the head, neck, ears, back, chest, pubic area, and groin
- live parasites fluoresce under Wood's lamp
- treat patients and known contacts by soaking hair in water-vinegar solution, applying permethrin lotion to skin, and washing all clothing and linen
- complications include secondary bacterial infections

MINICASE 147: PITYRIASIS ROSEA

An acute, initially plaque-like exanthem with no known cause
- occurs seasonally, clusters among contacts, and is more common in patients with atopy, seborrheic dermatitis, and acne
- presents with a 1- to 2-cm, scaly, pruritic, salmon-colored herald patch on the trunk, neck, or extremities followed by a secondary eruption of symmetrical lesions on the abdomen and thorax in a "Christmas tree pattern"
- skin biopsy is diagnostic
- treatment consists of zinc oxide, calamine lotion, topical steroids, and antihistamines, with refractory cases treated with systemic steroids, dapsone, and UV therapy
- recurrences are rare

MINICASE 148: PITYRIASIS VERSICOLOR

A common, benign, superficial cutaneous fungal infection caused by the normal skin organism Malassezia furfur
- presents with hypopigmented or hyperpigmented macules and patches on the chest and back
- diagnosis is usually clinical, although KOH scraping can confirm cigar-butt hyphae
- treat with topical agents (selenium sulfide or azole antifungals) or oral therapy with antifungals
- complications include recurrence and cosmetic disfigurement

Atlas Links: UCV2 MC-148   UCV1 M-M1-012

MINICASE 149: PYODERMA GANGRENOSUM

A large necrotic erosion with heaped-up borders commonly appearing on the shins
- idiopathic but related to ulcerative colitis, Crohn's disease, seronegative spondyloarthropathies
- presents with an acute-onset dark nodule that grows in size and then ulcerates
- treat the underlying disease

MINICASE 150: SEBORRHEIC KERATOSIS

An idiopathic, benign skin condition of the elderly
- presents with small brown or black skin plaques that appear "stuck on"
- no treatment is necessary
- may be removed with liquid nitrogen for cosmetic reasons

Atlas Link: UCV2 MC-150

MINICASE 151: TINEA CORPORIS (RINGWORM)

A dermatophyte fungal infection of the skin most often caused by the genera *Trichophyton* or *Microsporum*
- presents with pruritic, annular skin lesions with a raised, advancing, scaly border and central clearing
- KOH stain of scale shows fungal hyphae, culture is confirmatory and most commonly grows *Trichophyton rubrum*
- treat with topical imidazoles, treat widespread or refractory cases with systemic griseofulvin or itraconazole

Atlas Link: UCV2 MC-151

MINICASE 152: VITAMIN A TOXICITY

Most often iatrogenic
- presents with alopecia, skin scaling, orange discoloration, papilledema (pseudotumor cerebri), hyperkeratosis, and hepatomegaly
- x-ray of long bones and spine shows subcortical hyperostosis
- treat with moderation of vitamin A intake

MINICASE 153: VITILIGO

Hypopigmentation due to immune-mediated melanocyte destruction that may be idiopathic or associated with systemic autoimmune processes
- presents with patchy, symmetric skin and periorificial depigmentation
- Wood's lamp enhances chalk-white color, biopsy shows minimal inflammation and absence of melanocytes
- treat with glucocorticoids, UV therapy, and grafting

Atlas Link: UCV2 MC-153

ID/CC	An 18-year-old **male** presents with worsening **myopia** and **scoliosis**.
HPI	He complains that his schoolmates make fun of his **exceptionally long arms, fingers, and legs**.
PE	VS: normal. PE: slit-lamp exam shows **ectopia lentis** (lens dislocation); moderate **chest wall depression** (PECTUS EXCAVATUM); marked **scoliosis**; midsystolic click and soft 2/6 systolic murmur audible at apex with radiation to axilla; limbs long and thin with **increased arm span**; moderate **arachnodactyly**.
Labs	Normal.
Imaging	Echo: **mitral valve prolapse** with mild mitral valve insufficiency and mild **aortic root dilatation**.
Pathogenesis	Marfan's syndrome is an **autosomal-dominant** connective tissue disease that results from **a mutation in the fibrillin gene** (chromosome 15). Fibrillin is a 350-kDa glycoprotein that serves as a major component of elastin-associated microfibrils abundant in large blood vessels and the suspensory ligaments of the lens. **Cystic medial necrosis** of the aorta (predisposing to dissection) and **myxomatous cardiac valve** (usually aortic and mitral) disease are classical abnormalities.
Epidemiology	Occurs in 1 in 10,000 persons. Approximately 25% of patients have no affected parents; these are usually due to a new mutation. Occurs in **males** more often than in females.
Management	**Regular ophthalmologic surveillance** (follow closely for retinal detachment); **annual orthopedic consultation** to ensure early diagnosis of scoliosis; annual echocardiography to monitor aortic diameter and mitral valve function; **endocarditis prophylaxis**. Beta-adrenergic blockade to retard the rate of aortic dilatation; restrict significant physical activity to protect against aortic dissection. **Prophylactic replacement of the aortic root** with composite graft should be considered when the diameter approaches 50 to 55 mm (normal < 40 mm).

Complications Mitral valve prolapse typically develops early in life; aortic root dilatation can result in aortic regurgitation, aortic dissection, or aortic rupture. **Ectopia lentis** is a central diagnostic feature that results in severe myopia, cataract formation, ocular globe elongation, and retinal detachment. **Spontaneous pneumothoraces** secondary to multiple chest wall deformities as well as **inguinal and incisional hernias** are common. In untreated patients, mortality may result in the fourth or fifth decade due to aortic dissection or **CHF** secondary to aortic regurgitation.

Atlas Link   ☐☐☐☐☐ IM2-011

MINICASE 154: CHÉDIAK–HIGASHI SYNDROME

An autosomal-recessive defect of microtubule polymerization leading to impaired chemotaxis, degranulation, and phagocytosis
- presents with recurrent pyogenic staphylococcal and streptococcal infections
- decreased neutrophil count and large cytoplasmic granules
- treat with antibiotics appropriate to the infection

MINICASE 155: KARTAGENER'S SYNDROME

An autosomal-recessive disease of defective mucociliary clearance
- presents with chronic cough, recurrent sinusitis, primary sterility, and cardiac apical impulse in the right sixth intercostal space (DEXTROCARDIA)
- CXR shows dextrocardia, saccular and fusiform bronchial dilatation (BRONCHIECTASIS)
- EM shows absence of dynein arms within the cilia of sperm and bronchial cells
- treat with chest physiotherapy, antibiotics, bronchodilators

MINICASE 156: PORPHYRIA CUTANEA TARDA

An inherited or sporadic disorder of porphyrin metabolism, associated with alcohol, estrogens, pesticides, and viral hepatitis (HCV)

- presents with painless, fragile skin and blisters on the dorsum of the hands and forearms, skin hyperpigmentation, hypertrichosis, and dark brown urine
- increased uroporphyrin and 7-carboxylate porphyrin in urine, increased isocoproporphyrin in feces, increased total iron-binding capacity, and deficiency of liver uroporphyrinogen decarboxylase
- strongly associated with HCV infection
- treat with phlebotomy, alcohol avoidance, iron supplementation and low-dose oral chloroquine

ID/CC	A 40-year-old **male** complains of high, intermittent, spiking **fever with chills, right upper quadrant abdominal pain**, malaise, anorexia, and nausea of 1 week's duration.
HPI	He is a missionary who just returned from a 3-year stay in **rural South America**. Directed questioning reveals that he suffered from **diarrhea with blood and mucus** (DYSENTERY) as well as tenesmus on several occasions (due to intestinal amebiasis). He additionally reports a 4-kg weight loss over the past 2 months.
PE	VS: **fever** (39.3°C); tachycardia (HR 110); normal BP. PE: pallor; slight jaundice; no lymphadenopathy; right lung field shows **diminished breath sounds and basilar rales**; soft tissue edema and shiny appearance over right upper quadrant with **marked, tender hepatomegaly**; no ascites, spider angiomata, or caput medusae.
Labs	CBC: **anemia** (Hb 10.4); marked **leukocytosis** (18,350); **neutrophilia** (89%). Elevated ESR; **amebic trophozoites and ova in stool** (positivity rate is 10% to 30%); chocolate-colored ("anchovy sauce") pus obtained by needle aspiration of abscess does not show parasites (positivity rate is < 30%; amebae are confined to the periphery of lesion); positive complement fixation test reaction to *Entamoeba histolytica*.
Imaging	**[A]** US, abdomen: a large hypoechoic mass (1) is seen in the liver in another patient; note the diaphragm (D) and kidney (K). **[B]** CT, abdomen: a different case in which two areas of low attenuation are seen in the right lobe of the liver. **[C]** XR, abdomen: an air-fluid level is seen in this right subphrenic abscess (the normal gastric bubble is seen on the left).
Pathogenesis	Amebic abscess of the liver is a complication of intestinal infection with *Entamoeba histolytica*. A history of prior travel to an endemic area plus the triad of **fever, hepatomegaly**, and **right upper quadrant pain** are characteristics of hepatic amebic abscess.
Epidemiology	The liver is the most common extraintestinal location of amebiasis; prior intestinal infection may be asymptomatic or may present as amebic dysentery. The abscess is usually **single** and more commonly presents in the posterosuperior surface of the **right lobe of the liver**. It shows a **male predominance**.
Management	**Metronidazole** is the mainstay of therapy and is usually given with iodoquinol as a luminal amebicide. Dehydroemetine may be used for resistant cases and may be followed by chloroquine. Most abscesses will respond to medical therapy. Attempt **percutaneous**

aspiration/surgical drainage for imminent rupture, large abscesses, location in the left lobe (danger of pericardial rupture), secondary bacterial infection, or failure of medical treatment. Rule out hydatidiform disease (ECHINOCOCCOSIS) before attempting aspiration.

Complications **Secondary pyogenic infection** is the most common complication. **Rupture** may be life-threatening. Involvement of the psoas and gluteus muscle, pararectal spaces, spleen, or brain may occur by contiguity or metastatic dissemination.

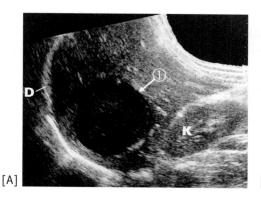

[A]

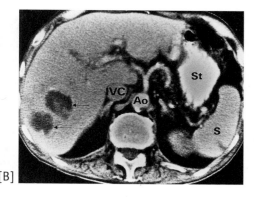

[B]

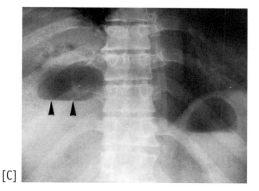

[C]

ID/CC	A 45-year-old man with bronchial **asthma** complains of a **productive cough**.
HPI	He also complains of progressively increasing breathlessness with intermittent attacks of severe dyspnea. He notes the presence of **brownish plugs** in his sputum.
PE	VS: **tachypnea** (RR 28). PE: mild respiratory distress; mild **cyanosis**; pallor; occasional rhonchi and wheezes heard bilaterally; **clubbing** of fingernails.
Labs	CBC: **eosinophilia**. Skin testing reveals immediate reaction to *Aspergillus fumigatus*; serum IgG to *A. fumigatus* present; serum IgE elevated; sputum culture grows *A. fumigatus*.
Imaging	CXR: branching, fingerlike shadows from mucoid impaction of dilated central bronchi involving the upper lobes (virtually pathognomonic).
Pathogenesis	Allergic bronchopulmonary aspergillosis is characterized by preexisting asthma accompanied by eosinophilia, IgE antibody to *Aspergillus*, and fleeting finger-shaped pulmonary infiltrates on CXR.
Epidemiology	Usually seen in atopic asthmatic individuals 20 to 40 years old.
Management	Allergen avoidance along with symptomatic management with **corticosteroids** and treatment of underlying lung disease (bronchodilators) are indicated. Systemic **antifungal therapy is not effective** in endobronchial disease.
Complications	*Aspergillus* may occasionally colonize a preexisting pulmonary cavity and produce an aspergilloma, which may be complicated by hemoptysis and should be treated by lobectomy. **Invasive aspergillosis** may occur in immune-compromised patients.

ID/CC A 28-year-old male is brought to the ER complaining of sudden-onset **double vision**, hoarseness, **slurred speech**, and **difficulty swallowing** for the past few hours.

HPI He also reports repeated vomiting and **symmetrical weakness** of the extremities that has **progressed caudally**. Directed questioning reveals that he ate some **home-canned stew** yesterday.

PE VS: **no fever**; postural hypotension. PE: **alert** but in acute distress; severe abdominal tenderness; bowel sounds depressed; ocular exam reveals **ptosis, dilated pupils sluggishly reacting to light**, and extraocular muscle paresis (type A may have no ocular signs); **DTRs depressed** in proportion to weakness.

Labs Blood positive for *Clostridium botulinum* toxin. PFTs: spirometry reveals normal vital capacity (to rule out respiratory muscle weakness).

Pathogenesis Botulism is an acute **descending paralytic disease** that **begins in the cranial nerves** and **descends caudally** to affect the extremities (without sensory deficits). Botulinum toxin **blocks acetylcholine release** in motor nerve terminals, resulting in a **flaccid paralysis**. Autonomic nerve endings may also be affected, resulting in dry mouth, constipation, or urine retention. Cases may be classified as **food-borne** botulism (derived from contaminated food), **wound** botulism (from localized toxin production), **infant** botulism (ingestion and/or gut production in infants), **adult-infant** botulism (similar to infants, but affecting older children and adults), or indeterminate. **Botulism should be considered only in afebrile, oriented patients who have a descending paralysis.**

Epidemiology Botulism occurs worldwide. Of the eight known types of *C. botulinum* toxins (types A–G), types A, B, and E commonly cause disease in humans. Food-borne illness is associated with **home-canned vegetables, fruit, and condiments** (infant poisoning is associated with contaminated honey). This type of botulism occurs when contaminated food is preserved with **spores** or when food is not heated to a temperature that destroys the **toxin**.

Management **Equine antitoxin** emergently while monitoring the patient for anaphylaxis and serum sickness. Emetic and gastric lavage may be useful if ingestion of contaminated food is recent. Infant botulism is not helped by antibiotics. Antibiotics that act at the neuromuscular junctions **(aminoglycosides) should be avoided.** Monitor spirometry, pulse oximetry, and ABGs to guard against

respiratory failure. If vital capacity falls $< 30\%$, intubation and **mechanical ventilation** are required, especially if paralysis, hypercarbia, and hypoxemia are progressing.

Complications Fatalities from botulism poisoning are low due to the availability of respiratory support. Artificial respiration may be required for weeks in severe cases, and residual autonomic dysfunction may be observed.

MINICASE 157: ACTINOMYCOSIS

Infection by *Actinomyces israelii*
- presents with abscess of the neck/jaw, abdomen, or chest
- causes classic draining sinuses with "sulfur granules"
- the disease readily crosses tissue planes and invades bone
- biopsy or smear shows branching hyphae-like bacteria
- treat with penicillin

Atlas Link: UCV1 M-M1-050

MINICASE 158: AMEBIASIS

Colonic infection by *Entamoeba histolytica*
- presents with diarrhea with mucus, abdominal cramps, and flatulence
- stool culture reveals causative protozoan
- treat with metronidazole or tinidazole, maintain hydration

Atlas Link: UCV1 M-M1-055

ID/CC	A 35-year-old male with **AIDS** complains of **diminution of vision** in his right eye.
HPI	The patient states that he sees **floaters** and acknowledges a recent **fever**.
PE	VS: **fever** (38.6°C). PE: funduscopic exam demonstrates **perivascular hemorrhagic exudates** and necrotic areas in right eye; decreased visual acuity.
Labs	CD4 count < 50.
Pathogenesis	CMV retinitis arises following **reactivation of a latent infection**, most commonly in AIDS patients with CD4 counts < 100. It causes progressive **necrotizing retinitis** that eventually leads to blindness.
Epidemiology	CMV is common; > 50% of adults have antibodies to the virus, and > 90% of homosexual men have **latent infections**. CMV retinitis is the most common opportunistic eye infection in HIV patients.
Management	Treatment may be local (to the affected eye alone), systemic, or a combination of both. Treatment options include IV ganciclovir, foscarnet, and cidofovir; oral ganciclovir; intravitreous injection of ganciclovir, foscarnet, and fomivirsen; and surgically implanted slow-release ganciclovir devices.
Complications	Retinal detachment and blindness, line sepsis from IV drug administration, and CMV involvement of the contralateral eye or other end-organ involvement (pneumonitis, colitis, encephalitis).

ID/CC	A 40-year-old male complains of **fever, cough, arthralgias**, and generalized malaise of 2 days' duration.
HPI	He also complains of left-sided pleuritic chest pain and mentions that he recently noticed a few **painful red lesions** on his shins. Three days ago he returned from a trip to the **southwestern United States**.
PE	VS: fever (38.9°C); tachypnea. PE: rales heard over left lower lobe; multiple tender **erythematous nodules** over both shins (ERYTHEMA NODOSUM); movements at large joints (knees and ankles) restricted by pain.
Labs	CBC/PBS: eosinophilia. *Coccidioides immitis* **spherules seen on sputum stain; coccidioidin skin test positive** (5-mm area of induration 48 hours after intradermal injection of coccidioidin).
Imaging	CXR: left lower lobe consolidation with hilar adenopathy.
Pathogenesis	The causative agent is *Coccidioides immitis*, a dimorphic fungus that grows in its natural soil habitat and on routine culture as a mold composed of **septate hyphae-bearing arthrospores**. The arthrospores are detached and swept into an aerosol that can easily be inhaled. Within the host, the highly infectious arthrospores mature into **spherules, the definitive tissue pathogen**. The spectrum of the disease varies from a primary pulmonary infection (whose severity varies from a mild influenza-like illness to severe pneumonitis) to a disseminated systemic form (more frequent in blacks and in pregnant or immune-compromised patients).
Epidemiology	The natural habitat of *C. immitis* is the desert soil of parts of California (e.g., **San Joaquin Valley**), southern Arizona, Utah, New Mexico, Nevada, southwestern Texas, Mexico, and Central and South America. The recent increase in reported cases has been largely due to the increased prevalence of AIDS, recent dust storms and earthquakes, and increased physician recognition of the disease. **Human-to-human transmission does not occur**.
Management	Mild to moderate disease **usually resolves without treatment. Amphotericin B** is the treatment of choice for critically ill patients; follow with oral **itraconazole** or **ketoconazole** for long-term suppression in HIV-positive and immune-compromised patients. Surgery may be necessary for chronic and progressive pulmonary lesions.

COCCIDIOIDOMYCOSIS

Complications Disseminated disease; chronic meningitis; skin lesions (maculopapular rash).

MINICASE 159: ASPERGILLOSIS

Infection by *Aspergillus* spp, most commonly *Aspergillus fumigatus*
- has three common presentations: allergic bronchopulmonary aspergillosis (ABPA, which presents with cough, dyspnea, fever, and bronchiectasis in chronic cases), aspergillomas (in which the fungus typically colonizes a preexisting cavity from chronic lung disease, tuberculosis, sarcoidosis, or emphysema and presents with hemoptysis), and invasive aspergillosis (bilateral necrotizing bronchopneumonia in patients with prolonged and profound granulocytopenia)
- in ABPA, CBC reveals eosinophilia and the serum precipitating antibody is present, whereas aspergillomas usually yield positive sputum cultures, and invasive aspergillosis is diagnosed on a transbronchial lung biopsy that demonstrates invasion with septate, acute branching hyphae and positive cultures
- CXR/CT reveal patchy, finger-shaped fleeting infiltrates and later central bronchiectasis in ABPA, whereas aspergilloma is seen as a characteristic intracavitary mass partially surrounded by a crescent of air, and invasive aspergillosis may be seen as a necrotizing bronchopneumonia
- treat ABPA with prednisone and bronchodilators, itraconazole and/or surgical resection for severe hemoptysis with aspergillomas, and amphotericin B/itraconazole for invasive aspergillosis

Atlas Links: UCV1 M-M1-059A, M-M1-059B, M-M1-059C

MINICASE 160: BACILLARY ANGIOMATOSIS

Skin infection caused by *Bartonella henselae*
- common in HIV infection
- presents with fever and erythematous papules resembling Kaposi's sarcoma
- treat with doxycycline or erythromycin

Atlas Link: UCV2 MC-160

MINICASE 161: BLASTOMYCOSIS

Pulmonary or disseminated infection caused by the dimorphic fungus *Blastomyces dermatitidis*
- presents with fever, weight loss, cough, and verrucous skin lesions
- diagnose by blood and sputum cultures, CXR with nodular infiltrates
- treat with amphotericin B

Atlas Link: UCV1 M-M1-065

ID/CC	A 35-year-old female presents with **delirium**.
HPI	She suddenly developed an **influenza-like syndrome approximately 1 week ago**. It has included **fever, chills, headaches, rigors, malaise, and cough**. Over the last several days, she has also developed a **truncal rash** and has become less coherent.
PE	VS: fever (38.7°C). PE: disoriented; **prominent maculopapular rash on trunk with several incipient lesions on extremities**; coarse breath sounds and rales bilaterally.
Labs	CBC: elevated WBC; normal hemoglobin, hematocrit, and platelets. **Weil-Felix test positive for antirickettsial antibodies.**
Imaging	CXR: bilateral patchy pulmonary infiltrates.
Pathogenesis	**Epidemic typhus is caused by *Rickettsia prowazekii*,** an obligate intracellular parasite that is **transmitted to humans by the body louse**. The disease begins when an infected individual is bitten by a louse, which ingests the rickettsial organism with the blood meal. The organism then multiplies in the gut of the louse. While biting another individual, the louse feces are excreted with *R. prowazekii*. The individual scratches, causing autoinoculation. One to three weeks after infection, the newly infected individual develops a flulike illness followed by a rash and signs of meningoencephalitis 5 to 9 days later.
Epidemiology	Epidemic typhus typically arises in times and places with **poor sanitation, crowding**, and **infrequent bathing**. Consequently, it has not been seen in the United States in more than 50 years. Among individuals who do contract the disease and are untreated, the mortality rate ranges from 10% to 60% and increases with age.
Management	**Tetracycline** (chloramphenicol second line). Prophylaxis depends on good **personal hygiene** and use of protective clothing in regions where typhus is prevalent. An inactivated vaccine of *R. prowazekii* is available abroad and for military personnel.
Complications	Myocarditis, intestinal hemorrhage, jaundice, renal insufficiency, vasculitis and thrombosis, and meningoencephalitis leading to delirium, coma, and death.

ID/CC	A 19-year-old male college student complains of urinary urgency and **painful urination** (DYSURIA) for the past 3 days.
HPI	He also complains of painful **swelling of the left side of his scrotum** (due to epididymitis). He notes that his underwear has been stained with a **thick, greenish, purulent urethral discharge** that is more profuse in the morning. He had **unprotected sex** during spring break **1 week ago** with a local striptease dancer.
PE	VS: normal. PE: erythema and swelling of urethral meatus with a thick, greenish-yellow, purulent discharge expressed; **left epididymis swollen, hard, and exquisitely tender**; normal prostate.
Labs	CBC: leukocytosis (11,500); 75% neutrophils. Gram stain of discharge shows **abundant PMNs** with **intracellular gram-negative diplococci**; culture in Thayer-Martin medium grows *Neisseria gonorrhoeae*; VDRL negative.
Pathogenesis	Gonorrhea is an STD caused by *Neisseria gonorrhoeae*, an oxidase-positive, gram-negative, intracellular diplococcus.
Epidemiology	Gonorrhea is a prevalent communicable disease in the United States. Its **incubation period varies from 2 to 10 days**; females are often asymptomatic carriers.
Management	**Antibiotic therapy** for uncomplicated disease consists of **ceftriaxone** (first line). Treatment should be followed by doxycycline or azithromycin owing to the **possibility of coexisting infection with *Chlamydia trachomatis*.** Complicated disease requires IV penicillin. **Treatment of sexual partners** is essential.
Complications	Patients may develop severe GU involvement and dissemination to virtually any organ or structure. Notable complications include PID with resultant sterility, **septic monoarthritis**, perihepatitis (FITZ-HUGH–CURTIS SYNDROME), and **ophthalmia neonatorum** in newborns.
Atlas Links	UCV2 IM2-018 UCV1 M-M1-091

INFECTIOUS DISEASE

GONORRHEA

MINICASE 162: BRUCELLOSIS

Caused by *Brucella abortus*, a gram-negative, aerobic coccobacillus transmitted to humans by drinking contaminated milk or direct contact with animal tissues
- presents with arthritis and undulating fever
- positive serologies and blood cultures
- treat with doxycycline and gentamicin or streptomycin

MINICASE 163: CHAGAS' DISEASE

A parasitic disease endemic to the Americas caused by *Trypanosoma cruzi*
- transmitted by reduviid bug bite
- presents in the acute stage with swollen eyelid from bite (ROMAÑA'S SIGN), ipsilateral auricular and cervical lymphadenitis, fever, and myocarditis
- the chronic stage presents with dilated cardiomyopathy (producing CHF and arrhythmias), megaesophagus (producing dysphagia and regurgitation), and megacolon (producing constipation)
- thick blood smear shows trypanosomes in the acute stage
- positive xenoculture, hemoculture, and serologic tests during the chronic stage
- treat with nifurtimox for acute disease

Atlas Link: UCV1 M-M1-071

MINICASE 164: CHLAMYDIA PNEUMONIA

Caused by *Chlamydia pneumoniae*
- presents with productive cough, few wheezes, and dyspnea
- CXR shows diffuse interstitial infiltrate
- treat with erythromycin

ID/CC	A 27-year-old **sexually active** male presents with **painful penile lesions**.
HPI	The patient also complains of **burning, itching**, and a **tingling sensation**. The lesions have progressed from erythematous to vesicular to ulcerated.
PE	VS: low-grade fever (38.4°C). PE: numerous **vesicular and ulcerated lesions on shaft of penis; inguinal lymphadenopathy**.
Labs	**Tzanck smear with multinucleated giant cells.**
Pathogenesis	The causative agent is HSV-2; usually acquired and transmitted through sexual or perinatal contact. The virus replicates at the site of infection before migrating up neurons and becoming **latent in the sensory ganglia (trigeminal and lumbosacral)**; exposure to sunlight or UV light, immunosuppression, infections, fever, stress, hormonal changes, trauma, and depression may cause reactivation. HSV-2 causes genital herpes, neonatal herpes, and aseptic meningitis.
Epidemiology	One of the most common sexually transmitted infections.
Management	**Antiviral therapy** (e.g., **acyclovir**, ganciclovir) for primary infections and to suppress genital recurrences. Foscarnet (IV) may be given for acyclovir-resistant cases or immune-compromised patients with systemic disease. Encourage prevention via latex condom use and cautious interpersonal contact with patients harboring active lesions.
Complications	HSV-1 is associated with encephalitis, herpetic whitlow (pustular lesion on the hand), esophagitis, and pneumonia. HSV-2 is associated with aseptic meningitis and neonatal herpes.
Atlas Links	UCV2 IM2-019A, IM2-019B UCV1 M-M1-100

MINICASE 165: COXSACKIEVIRUS INFECTIONS

Viral syndromes include hand, foot, and mouth disease and aseptic meningitis
- present with malaise, fever, flulike symptoms, and possibly hand and oral ulcerations
- there is no effective treatment
- complications include pericarditis and cardiomyopathy

Atlas Link: UCV2 MC-165

19   **HERPES GENITALIS**

ID/CC	A 72-year-old Caucasian male presents with a **painful rash** on the right side of his chest.
HPI	The patient has been taking medication for high blood pressure but is otherwise in excellent health. He also reports **severe burning pain preceding the appearance of the rash**.
PE	VS: low-grade fever (38.1°C). PE: unilateral vesicular eruption **confined to the right T6 dermatome**.
Labs	Tzanck smear of vesicle base reveals large **multinucleated epithelial giant cells**.
Pathogenesis	The causative agent is **varicella-zoster virus** (VZV), a double-stranded DNA virus of the herpesvirus family that causes two distinct pathologies: chickenpox (VARICELLA) and herpes zoster (SHINGLES). Chickenpox is a benign primary infection that is usually seen in children; herpes zoster results from **reactivation of the latent virus** and presents as a **dermatomal, painful vesicular rash**. When branches of the trigeminal nerve are involved, lesions may also appear in the mouth or tongue, around the eye (ZOSTER OPHTHALMICUS), and on the face. The precise mechanism of VZV reactivation is unknown, but it is thought that the virus remains latent in the dorsal root ganglion after a chickenpox infection; the dermatomes from T3 to L3 are most frequently involved.
Epidemiology	Herpes zoster can occur at all ages but primarily affects the elderly. Immunosuppressed patients are also at greater risk of more severe or disseminated infection.
Management	**Analgesics** for pain. **Antivirals** (e.g., acyclovir), especially in zoster ophthalmicus, immune-compromised hosts, and **HIV-positive patients**. Give antibiotics for overlying skin infections; steroids may reduce inflammation and pain.
Complications	Possible ophthalmic problems include conjunctivitis, keratitis, uveitis, and ocular muscle palsies; cerebral angiitis may result in focal neurologic deficits or ataxia. Other complications include postherpetic neuralgia and Ramsay-Hunt syndrome. Disseminated disease may develop in immune-compromised patients (particularly lymphoma patients).
Atlas Links	UCV2 IM2-020A, IM2-020B

HERPES ZOSTER (SHINGLES)

ID/CC	A 40-year-old **cave explorer** complains of **chronic dry cough, malaise, weight loss**, and **night sweats**.
HPI	The patient is also a chronic **smoker** but has no history of hemoptysis and has not experienced significant shortness of breath. The patient states that he grew up in the **Ohio River Valley** in the United States.
PE	VS: **fever** (38.5°C). PE: scattered rales over both lung fields.
Labs	CBC/PBS: anemia; leukopenia. Sputum culture yields *Histoplasma capsulatum*; complement fixation test for histoplasmosis reveals significantly raised titer.
Imaging	CXR: bronchopneumonia or multiple nodules are seen in primary form; apical fibronodular changes similar to TB in chronic form. XR, abdomen: calcification in the splenic area (seen in disseminated form).
Pathogenesis	The causative agent is *Histoplasma capsulatum*, a sporulating, dimorphic fungus that grows in soil (especially **soil enriched with the fecal material of chickens, starlings, and bats**); infection is acquired via **inhalation of spores** (due to aerosolization of fungus-laden soil). The organism has an affinity for fixed and circulating phagocytic cells of the reticuloendothelial system.
Epidemiology	Histoplasmosis is **endemic in the eastern-central United States**; the center of disease activity is within the Ohio and Mississippi river valleys. Although histoplasmosis has long been associated with farming and rural life, epidemic histoplasmosis has been increasingly reported among urban and suburban populations; the common denominator has been the disturbance of soil in and around a starling roost or accumulations of bat droppings.
Management	**Most patients** with primary pulmonary disease **do not require therapy**. Severely ill or immune-compromised patients and those with disseminated disease can be effectively treated with relatively low doses of **amphotericin B**.
Complications	**Disseminated histoplasmosis** develops rarely. Clinical disseminated histoplasmosis may present as a systemic illness with multiple-organ-system involvement that includes hepatosplenomegaly, generalized lymphadenopathy, fever, night sweats, anorexia, weight loss, anemia, and leukopenia. Adrenal insufficiency has been noted in 50% of these patients. In

21 **HISTOPLASMOSIS**

immune-compromised patients, progressive disseminated histoplasmosis is an important opportunistic infection. Chronic cavitary histoplasmosis affects middle-aged and elderly men who have severe COPD. Clinically, the disease is similar to cavitary tuberculosis.

MINICASE 166: CRYPTOSPORIDIOSIS

Caused by *Cryptosporidium parvum*
- presents as profuse, nonbloody, watery diarrhea, usually in AIDS patients
- acid-fast staining demonstrates oocysts in fresh stool
- treat with fluid and electrolyte repletion
- AIDS patients should boil their water at home to prevent disease contraction

Atlas Link: UCVI M-M1-081

MINICASE 167: ECHINOCOCCOSIS

A zoonosis produced by *Echinococcus granulosus*
- acquired by ingestion of food contaminated with dog feces
- presents with fever and hepatomegaly
- liver cysts can be seen on CT
- treat with surgical drainage
- complications include anaphylaxis resulting from cyst rupture

Atlas Link: UCVI M-M1-083

MINICASE 168: EHRLICHIOSIS

Infection by tick-borne bacteria of *Ehrlichia* spp
- presents with fever, malaise, myalgia, rash, headache, nausea, and vomiting
- can cause severe pulmonary and CNS disease
- leukopenia and thrombocytopenia
- serologic confirmation by elevated antibody titer on indirect immunofluorescence
- treat with doxycycline
- complications include seizures and coma

ID/CC A **15-year-old female** complains of **malaise, fatigue,** and loss of appetite for the past week.

HPI She also complains of mild **fever** and **sore throat**. Her boyfriend recently experienced similar symptoms that lasted approximately 3 weeks.

PE VS: mild tachycardia; low-grade **fever** (38.2°C). PE: firm, discrete, tender, nonmatted cervical **lymphadenopathy** and **pharyngitis** with marked erythema and a diffuse exudate; **petechiae at junction of hard and soft palate**; no hepatomegaly but **mild soft splenomegaly**.

Labs CBC: leukocytosis with >50% lymphocytes and monocytes. **[A]** PBS: >10% **atypical lymphocytes**. Monospot test for **heterophil antibodies positive**; specific EBV antibodies (EA, VLA, EBNA) also positive.

Pathogenesis The causative agent is **Epstein–Barr virus (EBV)**, a B-lymphotrophic human herpesvirus; it is transmitted primarily by **salivary contact** (as in kissing) and shed intermittently by all seropositive (clinical and subclinical) individuals. Infectious mononucleosis (IM) is defined as the **triad of pharyngitis, fever, and lymphadenopathy**

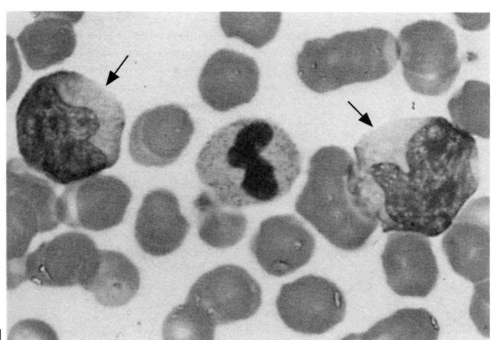

[A]

INFECTIOUS MONONUCLEOSIS

combined with **heterophil antibodies and atypical lymphocytosis**. A similar disease syndrome may be produced by other infections, such as toxoplasmosis, CMV, and HIV.

Epidemiology
Approximately 50% of the world's population has experienced a primary EBV infection before adolescence. Early infections are usually mild and subclinical, but a second wave of infection occurs at adolescence or adulthood that accounts for most cases of IM. The peak incidence of IM is 14 to 16 years for girls and 16 to 18 years for boys. EBV is associated with **nasopharyngeal carcinoma, Burkitt's lymphoma**, certain types of **B-cell lymphomas** (especially in immunosuppressed individuals), and hairy leukoplakia in AIDS patients.

Management
Supportive care, adequate bed rest. **Glucocorticoids** may hasten the resolution of pharyngitis and are indicated for airway obstruction, CNS involvement, marked thrombocytopenia, or hemolytic anemia. **Acyclovir, ganciclovir**, and **α-interferon** are potent inhibitors of EBV replication and halt oropharyngeal shedding; however, clinical benefits are minimal. Avoid contact sports for 6 to 8 weeks owing to the risk of splenic rupture. Also avoid antibiotics, particularly ampicillin, as it may cause a skin rash that can be a diagnostic clue to EBV infections.

Complications
Complications include hemolytic anemia, thrombocytopenia, Guillain–Barré syndrome, encephalitis, and splenic rupture with trauma. Airway obstruction may result from pharyngeal adenopathy. There is a strong association with Burkitt's lymphoma and increasing evidence that immunosuppressed individuals and bone-marrow allograft recipients may be predisposed to B-cell lymphoma.

Atlas Links UCV2 IM2-022   UCV1 H-M2-010

MINICASE 169: EPIDEMIC TYPHUS

An infectious febrile illness caused by *Rickettsia prowazekii*
- presents with severe headache, fever, chills, and a macular rash on the trunks and extremities with sparing of the face, palms, and soles
- positive Weil–Felix reaction, rise in complement-fixing antibodies for *R. prowazekii*
- treat with supportive care and antibiotics (tetracycline or chloramphenicol)

Atlas Link: UCV2 MC-169

ID/CC	A 76-year-old male presents to the ER with **confusion** and a **severe cough**.
HPI	The patient's illness began with the **abrupt onset of headache, muscle aches, and weakness** followed 24 hours later by **high fevers and shaking chills**. He subsequently developed a **nonproductive cough with pleuritic chest pain, dyspnea, nausea, vomiting**, and **diarrhea**. He is a chronic **smoker** and **drinks** heavily.
PE	VS: **high fever** (40.0°C); **bradycardia** (HR 50); tachypnea; normal BP. PE: disoriented; diaphoretic; **crackles bilaterally**.
Labs	CBC: **elevated WBC** (18,000). Lytes: **hyponatremia**. Gram stain of sputum reveals numerous neutrophils but no bacteria; **increased *Legionella* titers** by IFA. Culture on charcoal yeast extract medium positive for *Legionella*.
Imaging	CXR: patchy bronchopneumonia.
Pathogenesis	The causative agent is ***Legionella pneumophila***, a gram-negative aerobic bacillus that frequently resides in **environmental water sources**; acquired via **inhalation**. Infection is established in the presence of immunosuppression and/or impaired mucociliary clearance (as in smoking). Person-to-person transmission generally does not occur.
Epidemiology	**Older age, smoking**, and **depressed cell-mediated immunity** predispose to the development of this infection. The overall mortality rate is approximately 15%.
Management	**Erythromycin** is the drug of choice. Administer **rifampin in immune-compromised or severely ill patients**.
Complications	Dehydration, extrapulmonary infections, lung abscess, empyema, respiratory failure, pericarditis, endocarditis, myocarditis, shock, DIC, thrombotic thrombocytopenic purpura, peritonitis, renal failure, pyelonephritis, and pancreatitis.

INFECTIOUS DISEASE

LEGIONELLA PNEUMONIA

ID/CC   A 22-year-old military recruit presents with **altered mental status** following a bout of **high-grade fever**.

HPI   Three days ago the patient had reported that he felt ill and complained of **headache, stiff neck**, a severe cough, a sore throat, chills, and muscle aches.

PE   VS: **hypotension** (BP 82/40); **tachycardia** (HR 133); **fever** (39.6°C); tachypnea (RR 28). PE: **purpuric lesions** noted over axillae, flanks, wrists, and ankles; no papilledema.

Labs   CBC: **leukopenia**. LP: CSF with low glucose, high protein, and many PMNs. **Gram-negative diplococci** on Gram stain; platelet count and circulating clotting factors decreased; blood culture yields **meningococci**.

Pathogenesis   The causative agent is *Neisseria meningitidis*, a gram-negative diplococcus; spread by droplet infection and disseminated hematogenously from the nasopharynx. Produces the **Waterhouse–Friderichsen syndrome**, characterized by **meningitis, sepsis**, and **adrenal necrosis** (leading to fulminant vasomotor collapse and shock).

Epidemiology   Usually responsible for epidemic cases in the elderly population; however, any age group may be affected. A variable percentage of the population may carry the organism in the nasopharynx.

Management   **Aggressive IV fluid and steroid replacement** is key in vasomotor collapse secondary to adrenal failure. Administer ciprofloxacin or cardiovascular or respiratory support as necessary. **Penicillin is the drug of choice** in meningococcal infection; third-generation cephalosporins may be given for empiric therapy, and chloramphenicol for β-lactam-allergic patients. Administer **rifampin prophylaxis for all household contacts**. Vaccination is recommended for immunodeficient or asplenic patients, those traveling to endemic areas, and military recruits.

Complications   Fulminant meningococcemia with shock, peripheral gangrene, DIC, acidosis, brain injury (due to meningitis), and long-term adrenal insufficiency.

Atlas Link   ⓤⒸⓋ② IM2-024

ID/CC A 58-year-old male develops **pleuritic chest pain, fever,** and **shaking chills**.

HPI He also complains of a cough with **purulent sputum** formation. He is a chronic heavy **smoker with COPD**. He reports having had a **URI 1 week ago** with cough, coryza, and conjunctivitis.

PE VS: **high fever** (39.4°C); tachycardia (HR 117); tachypnea (RR 23); normal BP. PE: mild respiratory distress; **decreased breath sounds, inspiratory rales, dullness to percussion,** and **increased tactile fremitus** over right lower lung field.

Labs CBC: **leukocytosis** (17,500) with **neutrophilia** (84%). Elevated ESR. Lytes: normal. Sputum Gram stain shows **gram-positive diplococci in pairs** and many PMNs; sputum culture confirms *Streptococcus pneumoniae* (positive in only 25% of patients); blood cultures usually negative (positive in only 25% of patients).

Imaging **[A]** CXR: lobar consolidation in the right upper lobe bounded inferiorly by the horizontal fissure. **[B]** CT, chest: a different case in which an air bronchogram (1) is seen in area of consolidation (2).

Pathogenesis *S. pneumoniae* lung infection is a major cause of **lobar pneumonia** and typically affects those who are at the **extremes of age** or those who have an underlying disease. For example, asplenic patients are unable to efficiently clear nonopsonized bacteria from the blood.

Epidemiology Pneumococcal pneumonia usually follows a URI and is more common in patients with chronic cardiopulmonary disease as well as in sickle cell disease and asplenic (or splenectomized) patients, in whom disease is more severe. It is also more

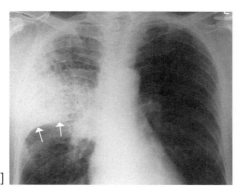

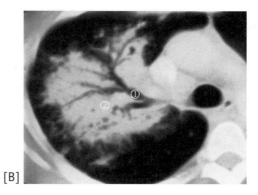

[A]   [B]

PNEUMOCOCCAL PNEUMONIA

common among smokers, renal-failure patients, alcoholics, and immune-compromised patients (HIV). There is a higher incidence in late winter and early spring.

Management Hospitalize if the patient is older than 65 years and has concurrent illnesses, is severely ill, or is homeless. Start empiric antibiotics based on likely pathogen. **Pneumococcus** is the most common cause of community-acquired pneumonia (CAP); **penicillin** is the drug of choice. For atypical pneumonia, *Mycoplasma* and *Chlamydia* are common pathogens; a macrolide is the drug of choice. For CAP requiring hospitalization, also consider *Haemophilus influenzae*, gram-negative rods, and *Legionella* as the cause; give second- or third-generation cephalosporin. For nosocomial pneumonia, consider *Pseudomonas, Staphylococcus aureus, Escherichia coli*, and *Klebsiella* as the cause; give empiric therapy with third-generation cephalosporin and aminoglycoside. Prevent with pneumococcal vaccine for patients who undergo splenectomy as well as those who have malignancies, sickle cell disease, or COPD.

Complications Atelectasis, bacteremia, meningitis, parapneumonic pleural effusion, lung abscess, pericarditis, and empyema.

Atlas Links ⬚UCVⅠ M-M2-035A, M-M2-035B, M-M2-035C, PG-M2-035

MINICASE 170: GENTAMICIN SIDE EFFECTS

Aminoglycoside antibiotics can cause nephrotoxicity (acute tubular necrosis) and ototoxicity
- presents with hearing loss, vertigo, and oliguric renal failure
- elevated BUN and creatinine
- granular and epithelial cell casts
- treat by discontinuing drug, giving IV fluids
- ototoxicity may be irreversible

ID/CC	A 23-year-old woman complains of the appearance of a **prominent diffuse rash** over the past 2 to 3 days.
HPI	The patient adds that about **1 week** before the rash appeared, she felt tired and had a **low-grade fever**, swollen cheeks and lymph nodes, mild nasal congestion, itchy eyes, and minor **joint aches** in her fingers, wrists, and knees. The rash **started on her face, spread to her trunk, and then spread down her arms and legs**, with each phase lasting about 1 day. She denies any sexual activity and denies the possibility of pregnancy.
PE	VS: normal. PE: **diffuse maculopapular rash; petechial exanthem on soft palate** (FORSCHHEIMER SPOTS) noted along with **patchy erythema** in oropharynx without exudate; mild nasal erythema without exudate; soft, movable **lymphadenopathy** noted in **postauricular** and posterior cervical distribution.
Labs	ELISA demonstrates **rubella-specific IgM and IgG antibodies** (acute rubella shows fourfold or higher increase in IgG titer). CBC: thrombocytopenia. Pregnancy test negative.
Pathogenesis	The causative agent is rubella virus, a **togavirus**. Transmission is via droplets shed in respiratory secretions, infecting the respiratory tract and, subsequently, the bloodstream, resulting in the characteristic rash, fever, and lymphadenopathy.
Epidemiology	Owing to greater than 95% seroconversion of vaccinated individuals, routine use of the live attenuated vaccine has virtually eliminated epidemic outbreaks of rubella among school-age children; **most cases now occur in young adults**. Although it is often subclinical, rubella is highly contagious, albeit less so than measles; it is transmissible via **respiratory droplets** from 1 week prior to the appearance of the rash to 15 days afterward, with the incubation period ranging from 14 to 21 days (average 18 days). Natural infection leads to lifelong immunity; antibody to rubella crosses the placenta and thereby protects the newborn.
Management	There is **no specific therapy** for rubella; the management of acute rubella consists of the **symptomatic relief** of fever (acetaminophen), arthralgias, arthritis, encephalitis, thrombocytopenia, etc. All infants should be **immunized with live attenuated virus vaccine** (the **first dose administered between 12 and 15 months of age** and **another dose given during childhood**). **Pregnant women should not be immunized**, and birth control should be practiced for a minimum of 3 months following

RUBELLA (GERMAN MEASLES)

vaccine administration. Consider therapeutic abortion if exposure occurs during pregnancy. **No serious side effects** have been reported after the administration of rubella **vaccine to immune-compromised** individuals.

Complications   **Congenital abnormalities**, which include early-onset cataracts, glaucoma, microphthalmia, hearing deficits, heart defects, and psychomotor retardation, occur primarily if the fetus is infected during the first trimester. Rarely, patients (adults more commonly than children) develop postinfectious encephalopathy that begins 1 to 6 days after the appearance of the rash.

Atlas Link   ⒰ⒸⓋ② IM2-026

MINICASE 171: GIARDIASIS

The most common protozoal infection in children in the United States
- transmitted through contaminated food or water
- presents as an acute or chronic diarrhea (bulky, frothy, malodorous, greasy stools) associated with crampy abdominal pain and flatulence, or may present as a malabsorption syndrome
- binucleate, pear-shaped, flagellated trophozoites and cysts found in stool or duodenal fluid sample
- treat with metronidazole

Atlas Links: ⒰ⒸⓋ① M-M1-089A, M-M1-089B

MINICASE 172: GRANULOMA INGUINALE

A chronic ulcerative STD involving the genitals and perineum caused by *Calymmatobacterium granulomatis*
- also called donovanosis
- Donovan bodies (dark-staining, encapsulated, intracellular rod-shaped inclusions in macrophages) demonstrated in crush preparations or fixed tissue sections
- culture of ulceration reveals the organism
- treat with Bactrim, tetracycline, or erythromycin

ID/CC	A 30-year-old male presents to the dermatology outpatient clinic complaining of a **generalized rash** and **hair loss**.
HPI	The skin eruption is nonpruritic. He reports having had **unprotected sexual intercourse** with multiple partners; on directed questioning he notes that he had a **painless ulcer** (CHANCRE) on his penis a few weeks ago.
PE	**Maculopapular skin rash** over entire body, including **palms and soles**; patches of hair loss involving scalp and eyebrows (FOLLICULAR SYPHILIDES); generalized nontender lymphadenopathy; mucous patches (silver-gray erosions with a red periphery) seen on tongue; **condylomata lata** (broad, moist, gray-white lesions) seen in perianal and intertriginous groin area; edges of skin are indurated (ELLIOT'S SIGN).
Labs	Darkfield examination of specimens obtained from condylomata and mucous patches reveals presence of treponemes; RPR positive; **VDRL titers increased** ($> 1{:}32$); FTA-ABS test (confirmatory) positive.
Pathogenesis	Causative agent is *Treponema pallidum*. Usually transmitted during sexual activity by direct contact with the mucocutaneous lesions that arise during the primary or secondary stage of syphilis (tertiary syphilis is rarely transmissible); however, vertical transmission from an untreated pregnant woman (maximum risk during 16 to 36 weeks' gestation) may result in congenital syphilis in the fetus.
Epidemiology	In the United States, the incidence of syphilis diminished markedly from the 1940s through the 1970s as a result of the introduction of antibiotics. Since then there have been two epidemics in the U.S.; the first, which occurred in the early 1980s and primarily involved homosexual and bisexual males, subsequently declined due to sexual behavior modification among this group in response to the risk of AIDS. The second epidemic, which occurred during the second half of the 1980s, primarily involved women, adolescents, and heterosexuals who exchanged sex for drugs or money. Approximately **one-half** of those involved in sexual activity with individuals infected with syphilis become infected.
Management	**Benzathine penicillin G** administered intramuscularly; if patient is sensitive to penicillin, erythromycin or doxycycline can be used. **Follow up with VDRL levels**. The CSF should be examined if the VDRL titer does not become negative or does not decrease

SYPHILIS—SECONDARY

dramatically in 6 months; if the CSF is abnormal, treat as for neurosyphilis. If relapse develops, patients should also be tested for HIV infection.

Complications   Tertiary syphilis, which includes neurosyphilis, Argyll–Robertson pupil abnormalities (afferent pupil defect), tabes dorsalis (destruction of posterior spinal columns), and syphilitic aortitis.

Atlas Links   ⬜Ⓤ©Ⓥ② IM2-027A, IM2-027B

MINICASE 173: HERPANGINA

An infection caused by coxsackievirus group A
- presents with sudden-onset high fever of short duration, headache, vomiting, myalgias, sore throat, and characteristic vesicular lesions on the soft palate, tonsils, and pharynx
- CBC reveals mild leukocytosis
- coxsackievirus A isolated from mucosal lesions
- treat with hydration, supportive care

MINICASE 174: HERPES LABIALIS

Herpes labialis is an extremely common contagious disease infection caused by the herpes simplex virus type 1 (HSV-1) and is characterized by the eruption of small and usually painful blisters on the lips, mouth, gums, or perioral skin
- an extremely common contagious disease that is transmitted through direct or indirect contact
- presents with itching, burning, or a tingling sensation for up to 2 days before characteristic vesicles filled with clear yellowish fluid appear on a red, painful skin area on the lips, mouth, gums, or skin around the mouth
- diagnosis is usually clinical, but a Tzanck test may reveal acantholytic giant cells
- treat with oral acyclovir (may shorten the course of the symptoms)
- complications include recurrences (secondary to reactivation), herpetic keratitis, and dissemination in immune-compromised patients

ID/CC	A 45-year-old male with a history of **untreated venereal disease** complains of **pain in his legs** and **difficulty walking**, especially in the dark.
HPI	For the past year, the patient has noted sporadic episodes of electric-like **"lightning" pain in his legs** that last for hours or days. He also complains of persistent numbness and tingling (feeling of "pins and needles") in his feet and has been **"stumbling"** whenever he turns quickly.
PE	VS: normal. PE: **discrepancy in pupillary size** (ANISOCORIA); involved pupil **reacts poorly to light but normally to accommodation** (ARGYLL–ROBERTSON PUPIL); cranial nerves grossly intact; motor exam 5/5 bilaterally throughout; DTRs 2+ and symmetric in upper extremities but **absent at patella and Achilles**; Babinski's absent bilaterally; sensory exam reveals **decreased vibratory and proprioception sense** in feet; **Romberg's sign positive**; patient maintains knees in an extended position; finger-to-nose intact bilaterally (tests cerebellar function).
Labs	CBC/Lytes: normal. PT/PTT and glucose normal; **serum FTA-ABS positive**. LP: **lymphocytic pleocytosis**; protein of 80 mg/dL; normal glucose; **positive FTA-ABS; positive oligoclonal bands** (FTA-ABS test is more sensitive and specific for the detection of treponemal antigens than VDRL).
Pathogenesis	Tabes dorsalis is a form of **neurosyphilis** that is characterized by **chronic progressive demyelination** of the posterior column of the spinal cord, posterior sensory ganglia (dorsal root ganglia), and nerve roots. *Treponema pallidum*, a spirochete, is the causative organism; it usually invades the CNS 3 to 18 months after systemic infection occurs.
Epidemiology	The incidence of latent syphilis is 7.4 per 100,000 in the United States.
Management	Treat with **IV penicillin**. If the patient is allergic to penicillin, he should undergo desensitization and then proceed with penicillin. Follow response to therapy by checking LP repeatedly over 2 years. Expect normalization of CSF VDRL by 1 year; relapse after 2 years of negative CSF is uncommon.
Complications	Complications include **Charcot's joints** (joint damage due to decreased sensation of lower limbs), incontinence secondary to

NEUROSYPHILIS (TABES DORSALIS)

neurogenic bladder, painless ulcers over pressure points, hearing loss, and visual loss due to uveitis, chorioretinitis, or optic neuritis. **Tabes crises** consist of abdominal pain and bladder dysfunction.

Atlas Link   ☐☐☐☐☐ IM2-028

MINICASE 175: HIV/AIDS

Acquired immune deficiency syndrome is caused by HIV, a retrovirus with a high affinity for CD4 T lymphocytes and monocytes
- acquired through sexual contact, IV drug use, blood products, perinatal transmission, and occupational exposure
- causes profound immunosuppression, rendering the host susceptible to opportunistic infections
- acute HIV presents with flulike symptoms of fever, sore throat, lymphadenopathy, diarrhea, rash, and weight loss
- acute illness is followed by a latent period in which the virus is held in check
- as CD4 count falls below 200, opportunistic infections (*Pneumocystis carinii, Mycobacterium tuberculosis, Mycobacterium avium*, toxoplasmosis, candidiasis, herpes zoster) may present
- CBC shows lymphocytopenia with a decreased CD4/CD8 ratio
- HIV is diagnosed with ELISA and confirmed with Western blot
- therapy centers on inhibiting viral replication (current regimens include two nucleoside reverse transcriptase inhibitors plus either a protease inhibitor or a non-nucleoside reverse transcriptase inhibitor), antimicrobial prophylaxis, and treatment of opportunistic infections
- complications include opportunistic infections, malignancies, and neuropsychiatric symptoms

---

MINICASE 176: HUMAN BITE

Usually due to closed-fist injury, chomping injury, or puncture-type injury resulting in direct bacterial contamination that is difficult to treat with normal cleansing
- physical exam reveals the bite wound, which may be overtly infected
- wound culture may reveal bacterial flora of the mouth and skin
- treat with ampicillin and tetanus immune globulin and/or toxoid
- complications include serious soft tissue infection, tendon damage, contracture, osteomyelitis, and cosmetic deformity

ID/CC	A 35-year-old **HIV-positive** male complains of **increasing fatigue, weight loss, fever**, and a **progressively worsening cough** of 6 weeks' duration.
HPI	He also acknowledges having **frequent night sweats**. He has no known contacts with tuberculosis but is known to have had **HIV infection** for 3 years; his last CD4 count was 150.
PE	VS: fever (39.5°C). PE: thin, lethargic; oral thrush; mild cervical lymphadenopathy bilaterally; mild rales audible in bilateral apices.
Labs	Sputum cultures positive for **acid-fast bacilli**; PPD and anergy panel nonreactive (secondary to immunosuppression); cultures eventually grow *Mycobacterium tuberculosis*.
Imaging	**[A]** CXR: primary complex with ill-defined right upper lobe consolidation (1) and right paratracheal adenopathy (2). **[B]** CXR: post-primary tuberculosis with right upper lobe consolidation and central cavitation.
Pathogenesis	The causative agent is *Mycobacterium tuberculosis*; infection is acquired **via inhalation of aerosolized droplets** that reach the lungs. The bacteria are then ingested by macrophages and are killed or persist and multiply. Organisms may disseminate to the lymphatic system and bloodstream until they are walled off by granulomatous inflammation (due to **type IV hypersensitivity reaction**). This process of primary infection is typically asymptomatic. Viable organisms remain dormant for years and may reactivate disease when host defenses are compromised.
Epidemiology	The incidence of tuberculosis continues to increase worldwide. The frequency of atypical presentations also continues to

INFECTIOUS DISEASE

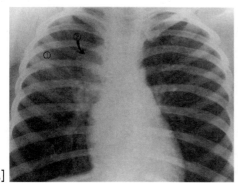

[A]

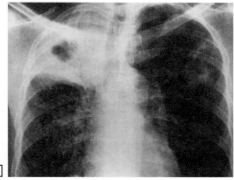

[B]

TUBERCULOSIS—PULMONARY

increase, particularly in the **elderly**, patients with **HIV** infection, and nursing home residents. HIV infection represents the most important risk factor for tuberculosis today, and the recent increase in the incidence of tuberculosis can be attributed to the HIV epidemic. Multi-drug-resistant strains of *M. tuberculosis* are now seen with increasing frequency.

Management   Immediate respiratory isolation. Start treatment with a **four-drug regimen of INH, rifampin, pyrazinamide**, and **ethambutol**. Directly observed therapy is an option for noncompliant patients. A presumptive diagnosis requires acid-fast bacilli on smear or a positive PPD in patients with CXR findings. A culture is required to confirm the diagnosis and to narrow antimycobacterial coverage. Five- or six-drug regimens should be used for outbreaks of strains resistant to INH and rifampin. Give supplemental **oral pyridoxine**, which prevents neuropathy due to vitamin B_6 deficiency caused by INH. **Serum bilirubin, liver enzymes, BUN**, and **creatinine** should be monitored prior to therapy. **Chemoprophylaxis** with INH or rifampin for 12 months should be given to high-risk individuals, close contacts of patients with INH-resistant tuberculosis, patients with positive tuberculin skin tests (< 35 years of age), and any of the following: known or suspected HIV infection, close contacts of newly diagnosed patients, recent converters, and patients with chronic illness. Immunization with BCG (results in a positive PPD) is widely used in developing countries where the incidence of tuberculosis is high, but is not used in the United States at this time.

Complications   Lobar or segmental collapse or consolidation, pleural effusion, pericardial involvement, tuberculoma formation, meningitis, and miliary tuberculosis.

Atlas Links   UCV1 M-M2-068A, M-M2-068B, M-M2-068C, PG-M2-068A, PG-M2-068B

MINICASE 177: INFLUENZA

Infection with influenza virus, transmitted via respiratory droplets
- presents with abrupt onset of fever, chills, malaise, cough, coryza, myalgia, and pharyngeal erythema
- CBC may show leukopenia
- viral culture of throat washings, complement fixation, and hemagglutination-inhibiting antibodies are positive for influenza virus
- treat with bed rest, analgesics, antitussives, amantadine
- trivalent virus vaccine confers partial immunity in most cases
- complications include bacterial superinfection, Reye's syndrome in children

ID/CC	A 24-year-old male complains of **persistent fever** of 2 weeks' duration along with mild **abdominal pain, constipation, a skin rash**, and a sore throat and cough.
HPI	He additionally complains of malaise, myalgias, arthralgias, and headaches. He reports having traveled to Mexico recently, where he ate **food** from **street vendors**.
PE	VS: **bradycardia** (HR 50); **fever** (38.5°C); normal BP. PE: confluent macular **erythematous rash on trunk** that fades on pressure (ROSE SPOTS); abdomen mildly distended and tender but with no peritoneal signs; mild **hepatosplenomegaly**.
Labs	CBC: anemia; **neutropenia**. Widal's test reveals **elevated "O" antigen titer** of 1:320 (> 1:160 is diagnostic); blood and stool cultures positive for *Salmonella typhi*. UA: proteinuria; various casts.
Imaging	CXR: normal (may show free subdiaphragmatic air in typhoid intestinal perforation).
Pathogenesis	The causative agent is *Salmonella typhi*. Typhoid fever predominantly affects human lymphoid tissue; the incubation period is variable (3 to 60 days) and is inversely proportional to the number of bacilli ingested. Infection classically results in **longitudinal ulcers in the ileum** (along Peyer's patches) and perforation (typically after 3 weeks of the disease), with subsequent peritonitis and variable patterns of GI bleeding leading to hypotension and hypovolemic shock.
Epidemiology	Typhoid fever has a worldwide distribution but is predominantly a disease of **developing countries** (due to poor sanitation); it is transmitted through **contaminated food or drink** (starchy foods, shellfish, eggs, and beverages, including milk), through **contact with the feces or urine** of patients or asymptomatic carriers (females with typhoid cholecystitis and patients with *Schistosoma hematobium* urine infections are frequently carriers), and by **houseflies** that may act as mechanical vectors. Typhoid fever is associated with significant morbidity and mortality approaching 15%.
Management	The primary antibiotic choices include **ceftriaxone** or **ciprofloxacin**. If the patient is in shock, administer **dexamethasone** before antibiotics. In the event of treatment failure or perforation, **laparotomy with resection** of the affected segment is

TYPHOID FEVER

indicated. Asymptomatic carriers may require cholecystectomy if they fail antibiotic therapy. Prevention involves hygienic/dietary measures; **typhoid vaccine** is advised for those traveling to endemic areas.

Complications Septic shock, intestinal perforation and bleeding, endocarditis, pneumonia, cholecystitis, and meningitis.

Atlas Link UCV2 IM2-030

MINICASE 178: LEISHMANIASIS—VISCERAL

Infection caused by *Leishmania donovani*, transmitted by the sand fly vector
• the disease is endemic in northeastern India, Nepal, and Sudan
• presents with ulcerating lesions in the skin and mucosa of the nasopharynx, darkening of the skin (HYPERPIGMENTATION), and massive splenomegaly
• CBC/PBS show anemia, leukopenia, and thrombocytopenia (PANCYTOPENIA), amastigotes in buffy coat, and Leishman-Donovan (LD) bodies on lymph node and splenic biopsy
• treat with sodium stibogluconate
• high mortality if left untreated

Atlas Links: UCV1 M-M2-014A, M-M2-014B, M-M2-014C, H-M2-014

MINICASE 179: LEPROSY

Protean infection caused by *Mycobacterium leprae*, most commonly causing disease in Africa and Latin America
• presents with peripheral neuropathies, rashes, peripheral joint and digit destruction, destruction of ear pinna, and hair loss
• biopsy demonstrates acid-fast bacilli
• treat with dapsone and rifampin

Atlas Links: UCV2 MC-179A, MC-179B

MINICASE 180: LYMPHOGRANULOMA VENEREUM

An STD caused by *Chlamydia trachomatis*
• presents with tender inguinal lymphadenopathy, a double genitocrural fold ("groove sign"), and painful genital ulcers
• inguinal node aspirate is diagnostic
• positive immunofluorescence test
• treat with doxycycline or erythromycin

ID/CC A 29-year-old **female** complains of **pain on urination** (DYSURIA).

HPI Directed questioning reveals that the patient has also experienced increased urinary **frequency** and **urgency**.

PE VS: normal. PE: mild suprapubic tenderness; no costovertebral angle tenderness.

Labs UA: **leukocyte esterase and nitrate positive; pyuria** without WBC casts; urine culture reveals $> 10^5$ CFU/mL (diagnostic for UTI).

Pathogenesis Most UTIs result from bacteria ascending into the bladder from the urethra. ***Escherichia coli*** is responsible for most (80%) cases of acute infections in patients without catheters, calculi, or urologic abnormalities. Other gram-negative rods, including ***Proteus, Klebsiella***, and ***Enterobacter***, are responsible for a smaller number of infections. Gram-positive cocci (e.g., *Staphylococcus saprophyticus*) also play a role in producing UTIs in sexually active women. UTIs are generally categorized as catheter-associated (usually nosocomial) or non-catheter-associated infections. UTIs may also be classified as those affecting the lower urinary tract (cystitis, urethritis, prostatitis) and those affecting the upper tract (pyelonephritis). Alkaline urine suggests the presence of a urea-splitting organism (most commonly *Proteus*).

Epidemiology The incidence of UTIs increases with the onset of sexual activity. They are more **prevalent during pregnancy** because of the decreased ureteral tone/ureteral peristalsis and temporary incompetence of the vesicoureteral valves. Ten to twenty percent of the elderly population and up to 50% of institutionalized elderly persons have bacteriuria.

Management Begin antibiotic therapy (**fluoroquinolones**) until the organism is cultured; then tailor antibiotics. **TMP-SMX is no longer** considered a **first-line** regimen owing to the increasing resistance of *E. coli*. **Predisposing factors** such as **vesicoureteral reflux, obstruction, neurogenic bladder**, or **calculi** should be identified and treated if possible. Recurrent infections should be identified to determine whether the same strain or a different strain is responsible for recurrence; patients with repeated infections or recent hospitalizations may harbor resistant strains. Individuals with recurrent infection (more than three

URINARY TRACT INFECTION (UTI)

infections per year) benefit from daily long-term administration of TMP-SMX. Recommend that patients urinate following sexual intercourse.

Complications   Treatment commonly results in complete resolution of symptoms. Lower tract infections are of concern because they can produce pain, discomfort, and lost time from work. Permanent renal damage may result with ascending infection and resultant pyelonephritis.

MINICASE 181: MALARIA

Plasmodium infection transmitted by mosquitos
- presents with high cyclical fever, fatigue, headache, hepatosplenomegaly, and thrombocytopenia
- plasmodia seen in erythrocytes on peripheral smear
- treat with chloroquine or mefloquine (in resistant areas)
- *Plasmodium falciparum* may lead to lethal cerebral malaria

Atlas Links: UCV1 H-M2-022A, H-M2-022B, H-M2-022C

MINICASE 182: MYCOPLASMA PNEUMONIA

The primary cause of "walking" or atypical pneumonia
- presents with fever, sore throat, headache, chills, and nonproductive to minimally productive cough
- associated with extrapulmonary manifestations such as bullous myringitis, cold antibody hemolytic anemia, erythema multiforme, and Raynaud's syndrome
- fourfold rise in complement fixation titer in paired sera, elevated cold-agglutinin titer
- CXR reveals patchy alveolar infiltrates commonly involving the right lower lobe
- treat with erythromycin
- complications include encephalitis, myocarditis, and hemolytic anemia

---

MINICASE 183: PROCTOCOLITIS

Infection of the rectum and colon, commonly by STDs following anal intercourse
- presents with severe rectal pain and blood or mucus per rectum
- endoscopic examination reveals erythema and inflamed rectal mucosa
- treat with doxycycline or Bactrim, sitz baths

MINICASE 184: PYOGENIC GRANULOMA

A polypoid form of capillary hemangioma that occurs as a rapidly growing exophytic red nodule attached by a stalk to the skin or gingival mucosa
- may be related to trauma or to the hormonal changes of pregnancy
- presents with a solitary reddish-brown nodular mass (2 to 3 cm) that may be ulcerated and tends to bleed easily
- biopsy reveals endothelial lined vascular spaces with acute and chronic inflammatory cells but no true granuloma formation
- treat with excisional biopsy
- complications include recurrence

MINICASE 185: Q FEVER

A zoonotic infection by *Coxiella burnetii*
- transmitted by livestock
- presents with fever and flulike symptoms
- CXR may show pneumonia
- diagnosis is made with serum serologies
- treat with doxycycline
- chronic Q fever can lead to endocarditis

MINICASE 186: SCABIES

A contagious disease caused by infestation of the skin by the mite *Sarcoptes scabiei*
- presents with intense itching that worsens at night and with papulovesicular lesions seen on the finger webs, hands, wrists, elbows, feet, buttocks, and axillae or nodules on the penile glans and shaft
- careful skin scrapings reveal ectoparasite under light microscope
- treat the patient and all family members with 5% permethrin cream or benzyl benzoate or with single-dose ivermectin when topical application is contraindicated

Atlas Links: UCV2 MC-186   UCV1 M-M2-049

MINICASE 187: SCARLET FEVER

Group A β-hemolytic streptococcal infection due to hypersensitivity to erythrogenic toxin
- presents with fever, an extensive erythematous rash, strawberry tongue, and pharyngitis
- culture of throat swab shows *Streptococcus pyogenes*
- ASO titer elevated
- treat with penicillin

Atlas Links: UCV2 MC-187A, MC-187B

MINICASES: 184–187

MINICASE 188: SHIGELLOSIS

Caused by *Shigella* enterotoxin, which activates adenylate cyclase
- presents with nausea, vomiting, and dysentery
- stool exam reveals leukocytes
- stool culture isolates nonmotile *Shigella* bacterium
- treat with rehydration and fluoroquinolones
- complications include Reiter's syndrome and hemolytic-uremic syndrome (following *Shigella dysenteriae* infection)

MINICASE 189: SYPHILIS—PRIMARY

An STD caused by *Treponema pallidum*, a spirochete
- presents with an indurated, painless chancre and inguinal adenopathy
- treponemes seen on dark-field examination of exudate from chancre
- VDRL positive, FTA-ABS positive
- treat with benzathine penicillin complications
- include progression to secondary or tertiary syphilis if left untreated

MINICASE 190: SYPHILIS—TERTIARY (AORTITIS)

Erosion of the aortic intima caused by tertiary syphilitic gummas leading to local dilatation of the aortic root or proximal artery
- presents with aortic regurgitation or can be asymptomatic
- FTA-ABS and VDRL document syphilis, US or CT demonstrates aortic dilatation
- management is surgical correction of the aneurysm and high-dose penicillin to treat the tertiary syphilis
- complications include aortic rupture leading to rapid hemodynamic collapse and death

Atlas Link: UCV1 PG-P2-045

MINICASE 191: TOXOPLASMOSIS

A systemic disease caused by the parasite *Toxoplasma gondii*
- acquired via cat feces
- common in AIDS patients but can be vertically transmitted
- presents with generalized lymphadenopathy, seizures, and cerebral abscesses (common in immune-compromised patients) and chorioretinitis (the most common manifestation of congenital infection)
- CT shows ring-enhancing brain lesions
- treat with pyrimethamine, sulfadiazine
- AIDS patients receive prophylactic Bactrim

Atlas Link: ⊞CⓋⓉ M-M2-065

MINICASE 192: TRICHINOSIS

Infection due to *Trichinella spiralis*, acquired by the ingestion of viable larvae in raw or undercooked meat
- presents with myalgias, fever, weakness, diarrhea, facial edema (mostly of the eyelids), and headache, but may progress to neurologic and cardiac involvement
- CBC reveals eosinophilia, elevated CPK
- muscle biopsy demonstrates free or encapsulated larvae
- treat with mebendazole and corticosteroids
- complications include meningitis, CHF, nephritis, and pneumonia

Atlas Link: ⊞CⓋⓉ M-M2-066

MINICASE 193: TULAREMIA

Caused by *Francisella tularensis*, a nonmotile, aerobic, gram-negative bacillus transmitted by contact with rabbits, squirrels, or tick bites
- presents with fever, ulcer, and adenopathy with suppuration
- diagnosis is made by direct fluorescent antibody staining
- treat with streptomycin and tetracycline

MINICASES: 191–193

MINICASE 194: ATOPY

Idiopathic propensity to IgE-mediated allergic reactions seen in asthmatics and patients with dermatitis
- strong familial inheritance
- presents with rhinitis, asthma, and eczema
- treatment is avoidance of allergic triggers, supportive use of antihistamines, bronchodilators, and topical corticosteroids

MINICASE 195: BEE STING

The most common cause of death from envenomation in the United States, bee sting can cause a severe anaphylactic reaction from toxin-mediated stimulation of mast cells
- presentation may range from localized pain and edema to urticaria, shortness of breath, anaphylaxis, and syncope
- treatment involves prompt stinger removal, administration of antihistamines, and emergent management of anaphylaxis if present (bronchodilators, corticosteroids, epinephrine, and vascular/respiratory support)
- complications include infections at sting sites, serum sickness, and rebound anaphylaxis

ID/CC A 19-year-old male on his first postoperative day after splenectomy experiences **marked oliguria** (< 20 cc urine/hr) and complains of **malaise, anorexia, and nausea.**

HPI He was found in **shock** after having been in a motorcycle accident. An immediate laparotomy was performed after rehydration, and a ruptured spleen with a **large hemoperitoneum** was found.

PE VS: normal. PE: well hydrated; **no suprapubic mass** palpable (enlargement of bladder in cases of postrenal ARF).

Labs CBC: anemia; **leukocytosis with left shift. Increased BUN and creatinine (BUN/creatinine ratio 10:20).** Lytes: **hyperkalemia; hyperphosphatemia.** ABGs: **metabolic acidosis.** UA: proteinuria; **renal tubular cell and granular casts**; urine specific gravity 1.012; urinary osmolality < 350 mOsm/kg; $Fe_{Na} > 1\%$; urine sodium > 20 mEq/L.

Imaging US, renal: no ureteral dilatation or enlargement of the kidney.

Pathogenesis Acute renal failure (ARF) may be oliguric (< 30 cc/hr) or nonoliguric and is classically divided into prerenal, intrinsic renal, and postrenal. **Prerenal ARF** is caused by a decrease in effective extracellular volume with decreased renal perfusion; it is associated with prolonged vomiting and diarrhea, acute blood loss (traumatic, GI, or gynecologic bleeding), fluid retention with heart disease (CHF), cirrhosis, drugs (NSAIDs, ACE inhibitors), vascular contraction, diuretics, and fluid sequestration (e.g., from pancreatitis, burns, peritonitis). Labs show muddy brown or hyaline casts, a BUN/creatinine ratio > 20, urine sodium < 10 mEq/L, $Fe_{Na} < 1\%$, urine osmolality > 500 mOsm/kg, and urine specific gravity > 1.018. **Renal** (INTRINSIC) **failure** is caused by prolonged ischemia (the most common cause of ATN, as in this case), nephrotoxins (cisplatin, **contrast media, aminoglycosides**), and diffuse renal cortical necrosis. **Postrenal** causes of ARF include any **obstruction to urine flow** from the kidney to the urethra, such as kidney stones, pelvic surgery, bladder or prostate tumors, retroperitoneal fibrosis, pelvic tumors, and urethral stricture.

Management Insert a **Foley catheter** and measure postvoid volume to rule out obstruction. If the patient is volume depleted, administer isotonic saline solution and wait for diuresis; if euvolemic, administer furosemide or dopamine. **Correct acidosis and electrolyte**

ACUTE TUBULAR NECROSIS—ISCHEMIC

abnormalities (hyperkalemia, hyperphosphatemia). Adjust meds according to creatinine clearance. **Dialysis** is indicated in severe hyperkalemia, pulmonary edema, refractory acidosis, fluid overload, pericarditis, and uremic encephalopathy.

Complications Complications include encephalopathy, GI bleeding (impaired platelet function), salt and fluid overload, pericarditis, severe hyperkalemia, hypocalcemia, increased anion-gap metabolic acidosis, and anemia. Opportunistic infections, poor wound healing, and muscle wasting occur due to the hypercatabolic state that is related to uremia and infection.

Atlas Links UCVI PG-P2-048, PM-P2-048

MINICASE 196: ADULT POLYCYSTIC KIDNEY DISEASE

Bilateral massive enlargement of the kidneys with multiple large cysts
- associated with polycystic liver disease, berry aneurysms, and mitral valve prolapse
- the mode of inheritance of the adult form is autosomal dominant, whereas that of the childhood form is autosomal recessive
- presents with pain, hematuria, hypertension, progressive renal failure, and SAH due to rupture of a berry aneurysm
- US reveals hepatic and renal cysts, carotid angiography reveals the presence of berry aneurysms
- treat hypertension, consider kidney transplant

MINICASE 197: AMYLOIDOSIS

Systemic deposition of one of several types of proteins within multiple organs
- can be idiopathic
- associated with diseases such as multiple myeloma or secondary to chronic inflammatory processes
- presents with dysfunction of multiple organs, including nephrotic syndrome, cardiomyopathy, hepatomegaly, and hypothyroidism
- biopsy demonstrates apple-green birefringence after Congo red staining of tissues
- treat the underlying cause (e.g., myeloma), consider organ transplant

Atlas Link: UCVI PM-P2-051

ID/CC	A 55-year-old female with gram-negative septicemia becomes lethargic and develops **decreased urine output**.
HPI	The patient was started on **IV gentamicin** 3 days ago. She subsequently developed increasing **confusion**.
PE	VS: low-grade fever (38.7°C); tachycardia (HR 110); tachypnea; hypotension (BP 90/50). PE: **disoriented; pericardial rub; asterixis**.
Labs	Lytes: **elevated potassium and phosphate. Elevated BUN and creatinine**; blood cultures reveal gram-negative bacilli. UA: **proteinuria; brownish pigmented granular casts with renal tubular epithelial casts in sediment; decreased urinary osmolality** (< 300 mOsm/kg); specific gravity 1.012; $Fe_{Na} > 1\%$. ABGs: metabolic acidosis.
Pathogenesis	Acute tubular necrosis (ATN) occurs secondary to an **ischemic or nephrotoxic insult**, causing focal tubular epithelial cell necrosis leading to **preglomerular vasoconstriction, tubular obstruction** by necrotic tubular epithelial cells and formed casts, and **tubular back leak**. Consequently, tubular flow decreases and intratubular pressure increases, yielding a lower GFR and ultimately oliguria. Oliguria results in **salt and water retention, hyperkalemia, uremia**, and a **metabolic acidosis**.
Epidemiology	ATN is the **most frequent cause of acute renal failure**. Risk factors are classified as toxic (**radiographic contrast, antibiotics, heavy metals, organic solvents, hemoglobinuria, myoglobinuria**) or ischemic (**decreased cardiac output, hemorrhage, sepsis**).
Management	**Correct the underlying etiology**; monitor fluid balance; restrict protein intake; discontinue offending drugs; correct electrolytes. If hypovolemia exists without evidence of obstruction, volume should be repleted in order to **maintain adequate cardiac output and renal perfusion**. After patients are euvolemic, start **diuretics** to promote urine flow. Uremic pericarditis, encephalopathy, severe hyperkalemia, and overt volume overload are indications for **peritoneal dialysis** or **hemodialysis**.
Complications	Renal failure in ATN often lasts 10 to 20 days, with **complete return to normal** renal functioning. Complications include fluid retention, hyperkalemia, anemia, infections, and uremia. Often fatal if left untreated.

33 **ACUTE TUBULAR NECROSIS—TOXIC**

ID/CC	A 44-year-old male with end-stage renal disease on hemodialysis complains of an **inability to move**.
HPI	The patient states that he **missed his dialysis appointment** 2 days ago. Since then he has experienced **progressive weakness**.
PE	VS: normal. PE: patient is awake, alert, and oriented ×3; lungs clear to auscultation; normal heart rate and rhythm; normal S_1 and S_2; 0/5 muscle strength in lower extremities with negative DTRs (FLACCID PARALYSIS); 1/5 strength in upper extremities; CN II–XII intact.
Labs	Lytes: **elevated potassium** (6.8 mEq/L). ECG: **prolonged PR interval and QRS duration; peaked T waves**.
Pathogenesis	**Intracellular potassium levels are approximately 150 mEq/L, whereas extracellular levels are ordinarily about 4 mEq/L**; an intracellular-to-extracellular shift may lead to profound hyperkalemia. Causes include insulin deficiency, acidosis, hyperosmolality, cell lysis, and succinylcholine therapy. Potassium levels are generally regulated by the kidney, so **derangements in renal function** (end-stage renal disease, aldosterone deficiency, aldosterone resistance) may also lead to alterations in potassium levels.
Management	ECG changes necessitate emergent **calcium gluconate** (minutes), **glucose and insulin** (20 to 30 minutes), and **sodium bicarbonate**. Stop all potassium intake. The next phase of treatment involves **potassium removal**, which may be accomplished with diuretics, dialysis, or cation exchange resins (Kayexalate). Potassium-sparing diuretics (e.g., spironolactone, amiloride) should be used cautiously in patients with chronic renal failure.
Complications	Failure to treat hyperkalemia leads to progressive cardiac dysfunction, ultimately leading to ventricular tachycardia, fibrillation, asystole, and death.

HYPERKALEMIA

ID/CC A 52-year-old man with rheumatoid arthritis and "borderline diabetes" presents to the outpatient clinic complaining of **abdominal bloating** and **bilateral ankle swelling** of several months' duration.

HPI The patient has suffered from severe rheumatoid arthritis for more than a decade and has been using **gold therapy** successfully for nearly 2 years. His blood sugar has been "borderline" for the past year.

PE VS: normal. PE: in no acute distress; no JVD; skin normal; lungs clear; cardiac exam normal; abdomen nontender and distended, with **positive fluid wave and shifting dullness**; extremities notable for **3+ pitting edema** in bilateral lower extremities to midcalves.

Labs CBC/Lytes: normal. UA: urine dipstick positive for 3+ protein but otherwise negative; 24-hour urine protein excretion 6.7 g/day (nephrotic-range proteinuria > 3.0 g/day). **Low serum albumin** (1.9 g/dL) and serum protein (5.4 g/dL); serum and urine electrophoresis negative; **hyperlipidemia**; renal biopsy shows **thickened glomerular basement membrane** and **"spike and dome" pattern** with silver methenamine staining; immunofluorescence reveals finely **granular deposits of IgG and C3** along capillary loops; subepithelial electron-dense deposits seen on electron microscopy; ANA negative; TFTs normal.

Pathogenesis The precise pathogenic mechanism of membranous glomerulonephritis is unknown; it is associated with a number of disorders, including hepatitis B, autoimmune diseases (SLE, diabetes mellitus, thyroiditis, multiple connective tissue disorders), and carcinoma, as well as with the use of drugs such as gold, penicillamine, and captopril.

Epidemiology Membranous glomerulonephritis is the **most common cause of primary nephrotic syndrome in adults**. Patients most often present in the fifth and sixth decades, and an increased incidence of occult neoplasms of the lung, stomach, and colon has been observed in patients older than 50 years.

Management **Prednisone** with or without cytotoxic agents for 3 months induces remission in some patients, but its efficacy is controversial.

MEMBRANOUS GLOMERULONEPHRITIS

Complications Slow but progressive loss of renal function over a period of 3 to 10 years may be observed in 10% of patients. Some patients may also develop secondary renal vein thromboses as a complicating feature.

MINICASE 198: DIABETIC NEPHROPATHY

Insidious proteinuria secondary to diabetic microangiopathy
- chronically progresses to glomerulosclerosis after approximately 10 years
- asymptomatic at first and then presents with hematuria, frothy urine (from protein), anasarca, and hypertension
- UA shows protein and fatty casts
- renal biopsy shows increased mesangial matrix and thickened basement membranes
- treat with ACE inhibitors, protein restriction, strict glucose control with insulin

Atlas Link: UCVI PM-P2-055

MINICASE 199: GOODPASTURE'S SYNDROME

Hemorrhagic alveolitis with nephritis, seen most frequently in young men
- caused by anti-glomerular basement membrane (anti-GBM) antibodies
- presents with hemoptysis, dyspnea, hematuria, and hypertension
- azotemia, oliguria, and hypoxemia; urine exam reveals proteinuria, RBCs, and RBC casts
- renal biopsy reveals necrotizing proliferative glomerulonephritis with crescent formation in > 50% of glomeruli (on light microscopy)
- anti-GBM antibodies found in the serum constitute the diagnostic marker for the disease
- immunofluorescence microscopy reveals characteristic linear IgG deposits in the glomerular basement membrane
- treat with plasma exchange, corticosteroids, cyclophosphamide, and azathioprine

Atlas Link: UCVI PM-P2-056

MINICASE 200: IgA NEPHROPATHY (BERGER'S DISEASE)

Idiopathic glomerulonephritis associated with upper respiratory or GI infections
- presents with hematuria
- normal C_3 and elevated serum IgA
- urine shows protein and red cell casts
- renal biopsy shows mesangial IgA deposition
- no effective treatment
- few patients progress to chronic renal failure

ID/CC	A **7-year-old** boy presents with a 2-month history of **lower extremity edema and progressive abdominal distention**.
HPI	The patient has no significant prior medical history, although he had a **"bad cold"** for several weeks that ended approximately 1 month ago. The parents deny any history of allergies, use of NSAIDs, photophobia, arthralgias, or myalgias.
PE	VS: normal. PE: in no acute distress; skin normal; no JVD; thyroid normal; lungs clear; cardiopulmonary exam normal; abdomen distended, with shifting dullness and palpable fluid thrill (due to **ascites**); extremities notable for **2+ pedal** and **ankle edema** bilaterally; normal skin exam.
Labs	CBC/Lytes: normal. Creatinine normal. UA: urine dipstick notable for 3+ proteinuria. **Serum albumin decreased**; serum protein decreased; **hypertriglyceridemia**; 24-hour urine protein 9.7 g/day (nephrotic-range proteinuria ≥ 3.0 g/day); serum and urine electrophoreses negative; ANA negative; following renal biopsy, light microscopy unremarkable; immunofluorescence negative for immunoglobulins; EM reveals **"fusion" of epithelial foot processes**.
Imaging	US, abdomen: excess peritoneal fluid (ASCITES).
Pathogenesis	The precise etiology of minimal-change disease remains unknown. It is associated with **recent viral URIs**, immunizations, hypersensitivity reactions to drugs (e.g., NSAIDs), or allergic reactions (e.g., bee stings) and may also occur as a paraneoplastic manifestation of Hodgkin's disease.
Epidemiology	Minimal-change disease is the **most common cause of nephrotic syndrome in children** but is occasionally seen in adults.
Management	**Prednisone** induces remission in 50% of adults and in 90% of children, but > 50% of patients relapse. Add cyclophosphamide or chlorambucil for relapsed disease. Although patients with minimal-change disease rarely progress to renal failure, they often develop complications requiring monitoring.
Complications	Patients have demonstrated increased susceptibility to bacterial infections (gram-positive organisms), spontaneous bacterial peritonitis, thromboembolic events, severe hyperlipidemia, and protein malnutrition.
Atlas Links	UCV2 IM2-036 UCV1 PM-P2-062

MINIMAL-CHANGE DISEASE

ID/CC A 73-year-old man with adult-onset **diabetes mellitus**, hypertension, and rheumatoid arthritis presents with a decline in **mental status** and **decreased urinary output**.

HPI The patient has been diabetic for nearly 30 years, with poorly controlled blood sugars despite insulin and oral agents; he has had **ocular disease** and **renal insufficiency** for > 5 years. He currently takes ACE inhibitors, a thiazide diuretic, and calcium channel blockers for hypertension and takes **NSAIDs** for persistent rheumatoid arthritis. He denies any asthma.

PE VS: no fever (37.1°C); tachycardia (HR 119); tachypnea (RR 28); hypertension (BP 140/84). PE: disoriented; lethargic, moderately responsive, and in mild distress.

Labs CBC: normal. Lytes: **hyperkalemia; hyperchloremia. Elevated BUN and creatinine.** ABGs: **non-anion-gap metabolic acidosis.** UA: **acidic urine** (pH < 5.5); **urinary anion gap positive;** proximal H^+ secretion normal.

Pathogenesis Renal tubular acidosis (RTA) results from deficient H^+ secretion in the distal tubule **(type I)**, defective bicarbonate reabsorption in the proximal tubule **(type II)**, and defective secretion of both potassium and H^+ in the distal nephron **(type IV)**. Type IV is due to a generalized distal nephron dysfunction attributable to either insufficient aldosterone production or intrinsic renal disease, causing **aldosterone resistance**; the resulting hyperkalemia decreases proximal tubule ammonia production and reduces H^+ secretion, leading to inadequate excretion of the acid load. These patients produce acidic urine despite reduced H^+ secretion because of inadequate ammonia to buffer the protons in the distal tubule. RTA is diagnosed by laboratory evidence of primary metabolic acidosis, a normal serum anion gap (< 12), a zero or positive urine anion gap, and exclusion of the presence of diarrhea, calcium chloride, or other acids.

Epidemiology Whereas types I and II RTA are rare, **type IV RTA is a common cause of normal anion-gap metabolic acidosis**. It is seen most commonly in patients with **renal insufficiency** and chronic medical illnesses such as **diabetes mellitus** (with nephropathy), **tubular interstitial renal disease, hypertension**, and AIDS. Drugs such as **NSAIDs, ACE inhibitors, and heparin** can also produce or contribute to type IV RTA.

RENAL TUBULAR ACIDOSIS

Management **Restrict dietary potassium; discontinue aldosterone antagonists** (NSAIDs, ACE inhibitors, heparin). Mineralocorticoid replacement with **fludrocortisone** usually improves hyperkalemia and acidosis but may worsen hypertension; patients with tubular resistance require higher doses, while hypertension and CHF are relative contraindications. **Loop diuretics**, sodium bicarbonate, and exchange resins can also be used. Acidosis generally improves as the hyperkalemic contribution to decreased ammonia production is corrected.

Complications Complications of type IV RTA are those of metabolic acidosis and hyperkalemia, including confusion, weakness, paresthesias, paralysis, arrhythmias, and even cardiac arrest when severe.

MINICASE 201: INTERSTITIAL CYSTITIS

A chronic abacterial bladder disorder occurring primarily in women
- presents with frequency, urgency, and suprapubic pain
- cytoscopy may show cystic wall inclusion bodies or ulcers or decreased bladder capacity
- biopsy to rule out dysplasia or carcinoma in situ
- no effective treatment

MINICASE 202: MEMBRANOPROLIFERATIVE GLOMERULONEPHRITIS (MPGN)

Idiopathic diffuse glomerular disease
- presents with anasarca, hematuria, and hypertension
- elevated BUN and creatinine, hypocomplementemia
- UA shows fatty casts, RBC casts, and proteins
- treat with aspirin
- renal transplant is the only definitive therapy

NEPHROLOGY/UROLOGY

ID/CC A 28-year-old white **female** presents to the clinic for a routine physical exam.

HPI On questioning, she notes that she has been urinating more frequently than normal and does not feel as strong as she once did (**polyuria** and **muscle weakness** secondary to hypokalemia caused by hyperaldosteronism).

PE VS: hypertension (BP 190/100). PE: thin and well developed; **loud, high-pitched, epigastric bruit bilaterally**.

Labs ABGs: **metabolic alkalosis**. Lytes: hypokalemia (3.0 mEq/L). Captopril test yields plasma renin activity of 22 ng/L/hr after captopril administration from baseline of 8 ng/L/hr.

Imaging US, renal artery (duplex): bilateral renal artery stenosis > 50%. **[A]** Angio, renal: a different case showing **"string of beads"** (alternating thick fibromuscular ridges and thin vessel wall) appearance of the right renal artery.

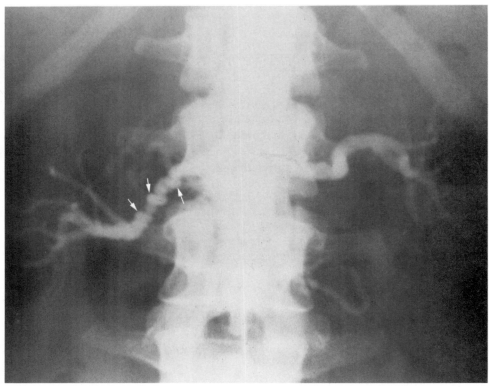

[A]

RENOVASCULAR HYPERTENSION—FIBROMUSCULAR DYSPLASIA

Pathogenesis Fibromuscular dysplasia is a **disease of small and medium-sized arteries** that is characterized most commonly by **medial hyperplasia with or without elastic membrane fibrosis** (MEDIAL DYSPLASIA). One may also observe periadventitial or intimal dysplasia. The stenosis thus produced results in decreased perfusion to the kidney, with subsequent activation of the renin-angiotensin-aldosterone axis. This hormonal activation results in hypertension (action of angiotensin II and volume expansion due to aldosterone) and electrolyte abnormalities secondary to hyperaldosteronism (hypernatremia, hypokalemia, and metabolic alkalosis). Polyuria may result from severe hypokalemia.

Epidemiology This disorder most commonly arises in **females** and **frequently affects the renal and carotid arteries**. It may, however, involve peripheral vasculature, producing symptoms similar to peripheral vascular disease. Rare in blacks.

Management Percutaneous transluminal angioplasty (cures > 50% of patients); medical management of hypertension (ACE inhibitors).

Complications Renal scarring secondary to ischemia.

Atlas Link UCV1 PG-P2-066

MINICASE 203: NEPHROTIC SYNDROME

A clinical complex characterized by proteinuria of > 35 g per 173 m^2 per 24 hr (in practice, > 30 to 35 g per 24 hr), hypoalbuminemia, edema, hyperlipidemia, lipiduria, and hypercoagulability
- six entities account for > 90% of cases: minimal change disease (the most common cause in children), focal and segmental glomerulosclerosis, membranous glomerulopathy (the most common cause in adults), membranoproliferative glomerulonephritis, diabetic nephropathy, and amyloidosis
- presents with lower extremity swelling, periorbital edema, and ascites
- renal biopsies show different patterns on light, immunofluorescence, and electron microscopy
- treatment varies depending on subtype
- in general, corticosteroids, cyclophosphamide, azathioprine, or cyclosporine may be used
- ascites is treated with fluid and salt restriction and diuretics
- renal transplantation should be considered for severe disease or for end-stage renal disease

NEPHROLOGY/UROLOGY

RENOVASCULAR HYPERTENSION—FIBROMUSCULAR DYSPLASIA

MINICASE 204: RENAL TRANSPLANT

Indicated for patients with end-stage renal disease when conservative treatment has failed and there are no reversible elements to the renal failure
- following a transplant, patients may present with complications related to organ rejection or immunosuppression
- clinically, acute organ rejection presents within the first 3 months with decreased urine output, hypertension, elevated creatinine, and leukocytosis
- immunosuppression is greatest within the first 6 months and accounts for the high incidence of opportunistic infections during that time, with CMV being a common pathogen
- key lab studies include UA, CBC, metabolic panel, and cultures
- complications include infection, graft failure, malignancy, liver failure, and hypertension

ID/CC	A 50-year-old woman presents after suffering a **tonic-clonic seizure**.
HPI	She also complains of weakness in the right arm and leg and has been experiencing a severe **headache, projectile vomiting**, and **blurring of vision**. She has traveled to **Mexico** within the last 5 years.
PE	VS: normal. PE: **papilledema**; motor weakness with increased tone noted in right arm and leg; DTRs exaggerated on right side; plantar response on right side is extensor; multiple nontender subcutaneous nodules noted over abdomen, arms, and neck.
Labs	CBC: eosinophilia. **Serum serology for cysticercosis positive**. LP (performed once elevated ICP is lowered): mononuclear cell-predominant pleocytosis; elevated proteins; low glucose.
Imaging	MR/CT, head: **multiple ring-enhancing lesions** involving the left cortex surrounded by considerable edema. XR, arm: multiple small soft tissue calcifications known as "puffed rice" lesions.
Pathogenesis	The causative agent of cysticercosis is *Taenia solium*. **Intestinal infection** occurs through the **ingestion of undercooked pork containing cysticerci**. Ingestion of *T. solium* eggs may also occur through consumption of **food contaminated** by egg-containing feces or by **autoinfection** involving hand-to-mouth fecal carriage. Clinical presentation depends on the organ compromised by the cysticerci; the most serious forms of cysticercosis are those with **ocular, cardiac**, and **neurologic** involvement.
Epidemiology	Most infections are encountered in **developing countries**, where intestinal *T. solium* infections occur frequently. In endemic regions, cysticercosis is the most common cause of seizure disorders.
Management	**Praziquantel** and **albendazole** are the mainstays of therapy. Give **corticosteroids** to limit inflammatory reactions to dying cysticerci; these reactions render ocular and spinal cysticercosis untreatable. CT scans should be repeated 3 to 6 months after therapy to evaluate cyst viability, and therapy should be repeated if viable cysts remain.
Complications	Seizures, hydrocephalus, and chronic meningitis.

39 **CYSTICERCOSIS**

ID/CC	A 32-year-old male is brought to the ER with **headache**, nausea, vomiting, and **fever**.
HPI	The patient is a former **IV drug user** who also complains of cough and shortness of breath. His next-door neighbor raises **pigeons** as a hobby.
PE	VS: **low-grade fever** (38.5°C); tachycardia (HR 146); hypotension (BP 80/55). PE: **altered sensorium; mild nuchal rigidity; papilledema**; oral thrush.
Labs	CBC: anemia; lymphopenia; decreased CD4+ T-cell count. LP: CSF with **lymphocytic pleocytosis**, increased protein, and decreased glucose. **India ink** preparation demonstrates round, yeastlike cells; **latex agglutination test for cryptococcal antigen positive**; HIV ELISA positive.
Imaging	CXR: lobar disease, pleural effusion, and hilar adenopathy. MR, brain: cerebral atrophy; no communicating hydrocephalus; **scattered focal** lesions.
Pathogenesis	The causative agent is *Cryptococcus neoformans*. The **most common opportunistic systemic fungal infection in patients with AIDS**, cryptococcosis is acquired via the respiratory route and disseminated hematogenously to the CNS. It most commonly affects the **meninges**.
Epidemiology	In the United States, half of all cases of cryptococcosis are found in **AIDS patients**; of those patients who are not HIV positive, most are **immunosuppressed. Pigeon droppings** and eucalyptus trees are considered significant environmental reservoirs.
Management	**IV amphotericin B** with **flucytosine; fluconazole** for maintenance therapy. Begin fluconazole after the CD4+ count drops below 100 cells/μL for candidal and cryptococcal prophylaxis.
Complications	With advancing illness, brainstem compression, coma, and death may occur rapidly. Pulmonary cryptococcosis may manifest as chest pain and cough; skin and osteolytic bone lesions may occur. Rarely, hepatitis, endophthalmitis, pericarditis, and endocarditis may occur. Acute renal failure may occur with amphotericin B.
Atlas Link	UCV1 M-M2-094

MENINGITIS—CRYPTOCOCCAL

MINICASE 205: VERTEBROBASILAR INSUFFICIENCY

Any interruption in blood flow to the brain stem, cerebellum, or occipital cortex, most commonly caused by atherosclerosis
- presents with vertigo, visual disturbances, facial numbness or paresthesias, dysphagia, dysarthria, syncope, or hemisensory extremity symptoms
- MR/CT to localize area of infarction
- treat with antiplatelet agents, thrombolytics, or anticoagulants, physical therapy
- complications include syndromes such as lateral and medial medullary infarction, basilar artery syndrome (locked-in state), and a persistent neurovegetative state with basilar occlusion

MINICASE 206: ALCOHOL INTOXICATION

Altered mental status due to alcohol ingestion
- presents with mood lability, impaired judgment, inappropriate aggressive and sexual behavior, nystagmus, ataxia, and slurred speech
- treat with thiamine, folate, and sedation as needed
- complications include withdrawal syndrome with seizure, agitation, and delirium tremens

MINICASE 207: ALCOHOLIC KETOACIDOSIS

Increased anion-gap acidosis
- distinguish from diabetic ketoacidosis by hypoglycemia
- seen in malnourished alcoholics
- presents with altered mental status, nausea, and vomiting
- anion-gap metabolic acidosis
- treat with IV fluids, thiamine, correct electrolyte abnormalities

ID/CC A 36-year-old man presents to the ER complaining of sudden-onset **pain and swelling in his left knee** of 3 hours' duration.

HPI The patient is a basketball player who reports having had **repeated arthroscopic procedures** on both knees. In addition to his sudden pain, he notes associated **fever and chills**. No other joint involvement was noted, and he denies any prior heart valve disease or intravenous drug use.

PE VS: fever (39.4°C). PE: back, hip, and ankle exams normal; left knee shows significant **induration, erythema, warmth, and marked tenderness to light palpation**; active range of motion limited by pain; passive range of motion intact; drawer tests negative.

Labs CBC: **marked leukocytosis** (> 100,000 with > 90% PMNs). Synovial fluid analysis shows **pleocytosis** (> 100,000 with > 90% PMNs) and **low glucose**; Gram stain positive for gram-positive cocci in clusters; culture reveals *Staphylococcus aureus.*

Imaging XR, knee: normal (normal early, but may manifest demineralization within a few days; complicating features such as osteomyelitis or periostitis may be seen as bony erosions or joint space narrowing within 2 weeks).

Pathogenesis Septic arthritis is characterized by **acute bacterial infection of a joint** accompanied by a systemic reaction with fever and chills, diagnostic joint fluid findings, evidence of concurrent infection, and response to antibiotics. Etiologically, it is classified as either **gonococcal** (causative agent *Neisseria gonorrhoeae*) or **nongonococcal** (most common causative agent *S. aureus*). Bacteria enter the affected joint via the **bloodstream**, having spread from a **neighboring site of infection** (e.g., bone or soft tissue), or by **direct inoculation**. Gonococcal arthritis, which accounts for up to half of all cases, is distinguished by prodromal migratory polyarthralgias, tenosynovitis, purulent monoarthritis, and a characteristic maculopapular or vesicular rash. Patients may or may not have accompanying GU complaints. Nongonococcal acute bacterial arthritis presents with sudden-onset monoarticular arthritis in weight-bearing joints with large joint effusions and occurs almost exclusively in individuals with known predisposing factors. Infections involving *S. aureus* usually arise after **surgery, penetrating injury**, or **other predisposing factors**.

Epidemiology Predisposing factors include **damaged joints** (osteoarthritis, rheumatoid arthritis, trauma, repeated procedures or surgeries),

persistent septicemia (intravenous drug users, endocarditis), **immunosuppression** (malignancy, HIV, end-stage renal disease), and **prosthetic joints** (loss of normal local host defenses).

Management Administration of **IV penicillinase-resistant β-lactam antibiotics** in combination with third-generation cephalosporin (e.g., cefotaxime or ceftriaxone) provides coverage for most infections. Local measures include hot compresses, joint immobilization (splint/traction), rest, and elevation. The drug of choice for gonococcal arthritis (based on joint aspirate Gram stain) is IV ceftriaxone. Patients with a high suspicion for gonococcal arthritis should be admitted to the hospital immediately to confirm the diagnosis and rule out endocarditis. Gonococcal arthritis responds promptly to antibiotic therapy within 24 to 48 hours, leading to complete recovery in nearly all cases. Nongonococcal arthritis also responds rapidly to antibiotic therapy in the absence of severe underlying disease. Patients are switched to oral cephalosporins or ciprofloxacin following clinical improvement for 24 to 48 hours to finish a 7-day treatment course. **Local aspiration** may be required with persistent reaccumulation of effusions. **Surgical drainage** is indicated with hip involvement (poor access by aspiration) or when medical therapy fails after 2 to 4 days. Early active-motion exercises may hasten recovery.

Complications Delayed or inadequate treatment may result in permanent articular destruction and bony ankylosis.

Atlas Links [UCV2] IM2-041A, IM2-041B

ID/CC	A 47-year-old male complains of **severe shortness of breath**.
HPI	The patient was admitted 2 days ago for acute pancreatitis.
PE	VS: **fever** (38.5°C); **tachycardia** (HR 112); **tachypnea** (RR 30–36); hypotension. PE: altered mental status; **central cyanosis**; warm, moist skin; accessory muscles (sternocleidomastoid and scalenes) used for respiration with intercostal retractions (respiratory distress); **bilateral inspiratory rales** and coarse breath sounds.
Labs	CBC: leukocytosis. ABGs: **severe hypoxemia** (< 70 mmHg) **refractory to increased FIO_2; ratio of PaO_2 to FIO_2 less than 200:1**. Swan-Ganz catheter reveals **pulmonary capillary wedge pressure < 18 mmHg** (noncardiogenic pulmonary edema); elevated amylase and lipase.
Imaging	**[A]** CXR: **diffuse bilateral alveolar and interstitial infiltrates** with normal heart size. Echo: **normal LV function**.

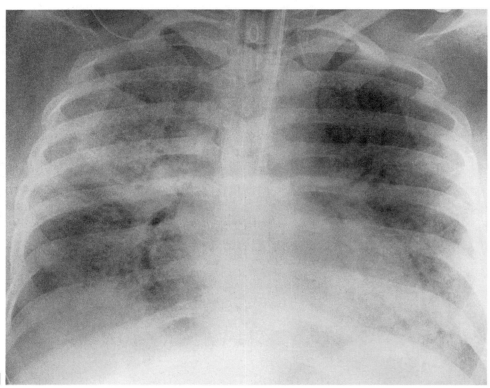

[A]

ADULT RESPIRATORY DISTRESS SYNDROME

Pathogenesis   Adult respiratory distress syndrome (ARDS) represents a common pathway for many pathologic processes (sepsis, shock, massive trauma, DIC, pneumonia, burns, oxygen toxicity, emboli) that lead to **increased capillary permeability** and consequent **extravasation of intraluminal contents into the interstitium and eventually the alveoli**, leading to pulmonary edema and atelectasis. The presence of vascular contents, especially fibrinogen, within the alveoli leads to **deranged surfactant production and fibrinolysis**, allowing for the formation of **hyaline membranes**. Eventually, this leads to **decreased lung compliance**, requiring greater inspiratory pressures, which translates into increased work of breathing.

Management   **Endotracheal intubation** and **mechanical ventilation** with positive end-expiratory pressure (PEEP) and **supplemental oxygen; IV fluids** for hypotension; DVT prophylaxis (SC heparin). **Nutritional supplementation** is needed because patients have an increased basal metabolism. **Antibiotics** for treatment of underlying sepsis.

Complications   Patients often suffer from multisystem organ failure, DIC, sepsis, or shock. ARDS ultimately leads to death in **50% to 60% of cases**. Patients who do survive generally recover 90% of their previous pulmonary function within the first year, but they may suffer oxygen toxicity secondary to long-term administration of $> 50\%$ FIo_2. Complications of PEEP include spontaneous pneumothorax and reduced cardiac output.

Atlas Link   UCV1   PM-P2-074

MINICASE 208: BRONCHIECTASIS

Dilatation of bronchioles secondary to chronic inflammation
- most commonly seen in chronic infection (e.g., tuberculosis, fungal) or cystic fibrosis
- presents with chronic productive cough, repeated pneumonias, hemoptysis, and crackles on exam
- CXR or CT reveals "honeycombing" and "tram tracking" due to bronchial wall thickening
- treat with aggressive chest physiotherapy, antibiotics for infection, and influenza vaccine
- complications include lung and metastatic abscesses and amyloidosis

ID/CC A 69-year-old white male who is a retired **shipyard worker** complains of a feeling of **breathlessness, initially on exertion and now even at rest**.

HPI The patient states that he worked for over **30 years in construction**, focusing primarily on the restoration of **old buildings**. He states that he has had a dry cough for years along with worsening fatigue, anorexia, and weight loss. He denies any history of smoking.

PE VS: no fever; tachycardia (HR 115); tachypnea (RR 30); normal BP. PE: clubbing; **dry end inspiratory fine bibasilar crackles**; loud P_2, parasternal heave (RVH) and JVD (secondary to pulmonary hypertension).

Labs Sputum examination reveals **asbestos bodies**. PFTs: **reduced total lung capacity, vital capacity, residual volume, and DL_{co};** normal FEV_1/FVC.

Imaging CXR: ground-glass appearance and small linear opacities (septal lines) most pronounced at bases. **[A]** CXR: large, irregular, calcified **pleural plaques** are seen bilaterally. **[B]** CT, chest: a different case demonstrates calcified pleural plaques, especially over the right hemidiaphragm.

Pathogenesis Asbestosis is a **diffuse interstitial fibrosing disease** that follows prolonged inhalation of any asbestiform fiber. Alveolar macrophages phagocytose these fibers and undergo membrane damage. Lysosomal enzymes are subsequently liberated, damaging the parenchyma of the lung, which heals by **scarring** and **fibrosis** and produces diffuse interstitial fibrosis. With advanced disease, the acinar units are eventually obliterated, forming a **"honeycombed lung."** Asbestos-related pleural disease is the most common manifestation of chronic exposure to asbestos and is completely benign.

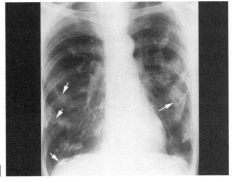

[A]

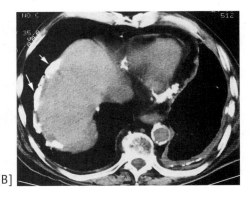

[B]

Epidemiology Asbestosis occurs primarily in individuals who have at least 10 years of moderate to severe **exposure to asbestos**, usually in the workplace (miners, shipyard workers, boilermakers, mill workers), and there is a 20- to 30-year **latency period**. Asbestos exposure is also associated with an increased risk of **malignant mesothelioma** (both pleural and peritoneal) and **lung cancer** (increased risk in chronic smokers).

Management There is no definitive treatment for asbestosis or mesothelioma; thus, pulmonary physiotherapy, **elimination of exposure**, and **smoking cessation** are crucial.

Complications Among patients with a history of cigarette smoking, the incidence of both **squamous cell** and **adenocarcinoma of the lung** is elevated approximately **55-fold**. Death usually occurs with onset of asbestosis-related symptoms within 12 to 24 months and may be earlier if Caplan's syndrome, pulmonary hypertension, or cor pulmonale develops.

MINICASE 209: CHURG–STRAUSS SYNDROME

Idiopathic systemic small- and medium-vessel granulomatous vasculitis
- presents with asthma and hypertension
- eosinophilia, elevated BUN and creatinine, and proteinuria
- CXR shows bilateral infiltrates
- treat with corticosteroids

MINICASE 210: HYPERSENSITIVITY PNEUMONITIS

An interstitial lung disease that results from inhalation of organic antigens
- presents with dyspnea, fatigue, dry cough, and fine rales
- CXR shows reticulonodular infiltrates
- PFTs show restrictive pattern
- treat with corticosteroids, avoidance of offending agent

ID/CC	A 30-year-old man presents to the emergency room with an acute attack of **shortness of breath, coughing**, and **wheezing**.
HPI	The patient states that the attack occurred several hours after he played with a neighbor's **cat**. Review of systems is positive for **allergic rhinitis, postnasal drip, atopic dermatitis**, and **GERD**.
PE	VS: no fever; **tachycardia** (HR 130); **tachypnea** (RR 40); **pulsus paradoxus**. PE: **confused** and **diaphoretic; uses accessory muscles** of respiration; cyanosis; lungs hyperresonant to percussion; inspiratory and expiratory **diffuse wheezing** bilaterally; increased E:I ratio.
Labs	CBC: **eosinophilia**. ABGs: primary **respiratory alkalosis** with **reduced PO_2 and PCO_2** (elevated PCO_2 indicates respiratory failure); **peak flows decreased**. PFTs: low **FEV_1/FVC** with > 15% improvement of FEV_1 following administration of β_2-agonist; sputum analysis reveals **Curschmann's spirals** (mucus that forms casts in small airways) and **Charcot–Leyden crystals** (eosinophil breakdown products); elevated serum IgE.
Imaging	CXR: hyperinflation, flattened diaphragms (secondary to air trapping and increased residual volume).
Pathogenesis	Bronchial asthma is characterized by airway constriction secondary to reversible, episodic contractions of airway smooth muscle due to **hyperreactivity**, hypersecretion of **tenacious mucus**, and **mucosal edema** (due to inflammation). It may occur as a response to an allergen **(type I hypersensitivity reaction)** or may be **intrinsic**. Acute attacks may be precipitated by cold air or pollution, smoking, airway infections, emotional stress, and exercise.
Epidemiology	Afflicts 4% to 5% of the population. Children often have the **atopic** form (which may remit in the second decade), whereas intrinsic and occupational asthma arise more commonly in adults.
Management	**Prophylaxis with inhaled corticosteroids** (beclomethasone), cromolyn sodium (particularly in children with extrinsic asthma), **leukotriene inhibitors**, and, in severe cases, oral steroids. In acute attacks, give **albuterol** and ipratropium for bronchodilation. Severe episodes may necessitate hospital admission, **IV corticosteroids**, and intubation for respiratory failure.

ASTHMA, CHRONIC

Complications Asthma may lead to **unremitting bronchospasm** (status asthmaticus), **respiratory failure**, respiratory arrest, and death. Patients are also prone to develop recurrent respiratory infections and pneumothorax.

MINICASE 211: INTERSTITIAL LUNG DISEASE

Inflammation and fibrosis of the interalveolar spaces of the lung
- can be idiopathic or secondary to granulomatous disease, toxic inhalations, particulate toxins (e.g., asbestos, silica), or collagen vascular disease
- presents with acute or chronic progression of dyspnea and exercise intolerance
- CXR reveals classic "honeycomb" appearance of the lung
- spirometry reveals restrictive pathology (proportionately reduced FEV_1 and FVC, hence normal FEV_1/FVC)
- treatment is directed at the underlying cause; supplemental oxygen
- complications include pulmonary hypertension leading to cor pulmonale

---

MINICASE 212: LÖFFLER'S SYNDROME

Eosinophilic pneumonia caused by drugs or parasitic infection
- presents with fever, cough, and dyspnea
- peripheral blood eosinophilia
- pulmonary infiltrates on CXR
- remove offending drug or treat parasitic infection, give corticosteroids if no cause is found

---

MINICASE 213: LUNG TRANSPLANT

Indicated for patients with nonmalignant pulmonary disease (pulmonary fibrosis, cystic fibrosis, chronic emphysema, α_1-antitrypsin deficiency, and silicosis) who are unresponsive to conventional treatment and who have a life expectancy of < 1 year
- transplant is grafted just superior to the bifurcation at the carina
- current survival rates are 75% to 90% for 1 year and $> 50\%$ beyond 2 years
- complications include those of the pleural space (pneumothorax, hemothorax, chylothorax, empyema), those of the lung parenchyma (acute rejection, pulmonary embolism), opportunistic infections that are common in the early postoperative period (bacterial, viral, fungal, parasitic), and immunosuppression-related complications (often GI, hematologic, and hepatobiliary)

ID/CC	A 56-year-old male presents with **shortness of breath** and a **chronic cough** productive of **copious mucoid sputum**.
HPI	Over the **past 3 years**, his symptoms have occurred for at least 3 months out of every year. He also reports a 40-pack-year **smoking history**.
PE	VS: **tachypnea** (RR 25). PE: **blue lips** (CENTRAL CYANOSIS); plethora; bilateral rhonchi and wheezes.
Labs	CBC: hematocrit increased. ABGs: **hypoxia** and **hypercapnia**. ECG: presence of P-pulmonale and poor progression of R wave in chest leads. PFTs: **obstructive** pattern of increased residual volume and decreased FEV_1/FVC.
Imaging	CXR, PA: presence of increased basilar bronchovascular markings and thickened bronchial walls.
Pathogenesis	The pathologic hallmark of chronic bronchitis is **enlargement of the mucous glands** in the major bronchi. The diameter of the mucous glands relative to the thickness of the bronchial wall (the Reid index) is typically increased from values of 0.26 to 0.44 in healthy persons to > 0.50 in patients with chronic bronchitis. **Smoking** and **occupational exposure** to harmful substances are the principal etiologic factors.
Epidemiology	Seen primarily in smokers.
Management	**Smoking cessation** and long-term administration of **supplemental oxygen** are the two most important interventions. **Bronchodilators, antibiotics, and corticosteroids** may be used in acute exacerbations.
Complications	**Cor pulmonale**.

COPD—CHRONIC BRONCHITIS

ID/CC A 60-year-old male complains of progressive **shortness of breath on exertion** and a **nonproductive cough**.

HPI He has a 60-pack-year **smoking history**.

PE VS: no fever; **tachypnea** (RR 24). PE: moderate **respiratory distress; pursed lips**; using **accessory muscles** of respiration; **barrel-shaped chest; hyperresonant percussion** note; distant breath sounds; scattered rhonchi heard bilaterally on auscultation; heart sounds distant.

Labs ABGs: mild hypoxia with hypocapnia. PFTs: **decreased FEV_1/FVC ratio**; decreased DL_{co}; increased TLC, FRC, and RV.

Imaging **[A]** CXR, PA: hypertranslucent lung fields with large bullae (1); flattening of the diaphragm (2) and elongated tubular heart shadow. **[B]** CT, chest: multiple large bullae (1). **[C]** CT, chest: innumerable smaller bullae.

Pathogenesis Emphysema is abnormal permanent **enlargement of air spaces distal to the terminal bronchiole** accompanied by the **destruction of the alveolar walls**. It may involve the acinus and the lobule

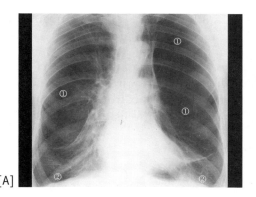

[A]

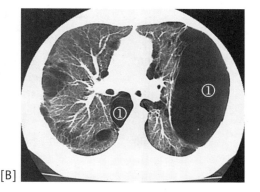

[B]

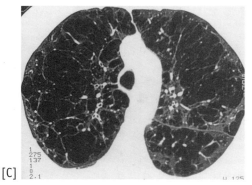

[C]

COPD—EMPHYSEMA

uniformly (panacinar) or may primarily involve the respiratory bronchioles (centriacinar). **Panacinar** emphysema is common in patients with α_1-**antitrypsin** deficiency. Typically, the lower lobes show more involvement than the upper lobes. **Centriacinar** emphysema is commonly found in **cigarette smokers** and is rare in nonsmokers. It is usually more extensive and severe in the upper lobes. Emphysema leads to a **reduction in elastic recoil** in the lung that leads to narrowing of the airways with a subsequent decrease in expiratory flow rates (airway obstruction).

Epidemiology Chronic airway obstruction (CAO) is a leading cause of death in the United States and is second only to CAD as a Social Security-compensated disability. From **80% to 90% of cases of CAO can be attributed to cigarette smoking**; a small percentage is attributable to α_1-**antitrypsin deficiency**. The risk of death from emphysema or chronic bronchitis is 30 times greater for heavy smokers (> 25 cigarettes/day) than for nonsmokers.

Management **Smoking cessation** and long-term administration of **supplemental oxygen** are the two most important interventions. **Bronchodilators** are commonly used; **antibiotics** in acute exacerbations; **corticosteroids** in resistant cases. Influenza and pneumococcal vaccines are recommended. Lung volume reduction surgery and lung transplantation are promising treatments. Surgical excision of bullae may be necessary to provide relief.

Complications Chronic hypoxemia causes **secondary erythrocytosis** and contributes to exercise limitation, pulmonary hypertension, right heart failure, spontaneous pneumothorax from rupturing of blebs and bullae, and impaired neuropsychiatric function.

Atlas Links UCV1 PG-P2-081, PM-P2-081

MINICASE 214: PRIMARY PULMONARY HYPERTENSION

An idiopathic increase in pulmonary artery pressure and pulmonary vascular resistance, seen in young women
- presents with progressive dyspnea refractory to oxygen therapy, large "a" wave in JVP, and loud P2
- polycythemia
- ECG shows right axis deviation and right ventricular and atrial hypertrophy
- treat with prostacyclin, calcium channel blockers, adenosine or nitric oxide
- consider heart-lung transplantation, without which the disease progresses to cor pulmonale

Atlas Link: UCV1 PG-P2-090

ID/CC A **28-year-old man** presents to the outpatient clinic with complaints of **acute-onset** right-sided **chest pain** and **shortness of breath** that started yesterday afternoon.

HPI The pain and dyspnea are localized to the right side, are unrelated to position or activity, and actually started while the patient was resting. His symptoms have been stable over the past day, and he has had no progressive difficulty breathing. He has no prior medical or family history but reports that he has **smoked** approximately one pack of cigarettes per day for 7 years.

PE VS: mild tachycardia. PE: **tall and thin**; in mild distress; no JVD or lymphadenopathy; **diminished breath sounds, decreased tactile fremitus**, and **hyperresonance** in right lung fields; no mediastinal or tracheal shift or cyanosis noted; cardiac exam normal.

Labs ABGs: **hypoxemia**, acute respiratory alkalosis. ECG: unremarkable.

Imaging **[A]** and **[B]** CXR: the diagnostic **visceral pleural line** is seen on the right side; peripheral to this, the area is seen to be **hyperlucent**, as the lung has retracted.

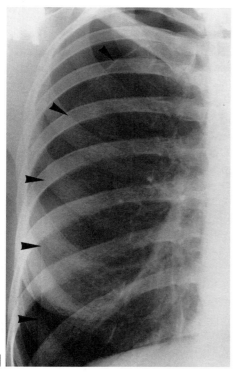

[A]

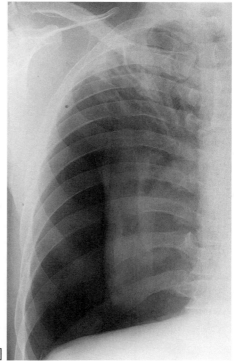

[B]

PNEUMOTHORAX—SPONTANEOUS

Pathogenesis   Pneumothorax represents an accumulation of air in the pleural space and is classified as spontaneous or traumatic. It is believed to occur as a result of the **rupture of subpleural apical blebs** in response to **high negative intrapleural pressure**. Spontaneous pneumothorax is most commonly primary (without an underlying cause) but may be secondary to preexisting pulmonary disease (COPD, asthma, cystic fibrosis, TB) and occurs predominantly in smokers. Traumatic pneumothorax results from penetrating or nonpenetrating trauma, often from iatrogenic causes (e.g., thoracocentesis, pleural biopsy, positive-pressure mechanical ventilation).

Epidemiology   Pneumothorax typically affects **tall, thin men** in their **third and fourth decades**. Prior history of *Pneumocystis carinii* pneumonia and use of aerosolized pentamidine are particularly notable risk factors for pneumothorax.

Management   Patients with a small new pneumothorax should be hospitalized, placed on bed rest, given oxygen, and monitored with serial chest x-rays. Small pneumothoraces often resolve spontaneously but may progress unpredictably to tension pneumothorax, which is treated by immediate insertion of a large-bore needle in the affected side, followed by **tube thoracostomy**. Patients with tension or secondary pneumothorax, those with severe symptoms, or those with a large pneumothorax should undergo **chest tube placement** (tube thoracostomy). The chest tube is placed to water-seal suction until the lung begins to expand. Air leaks, recurrence, and pulmonary edema may occur. Patients should be advised to **stop smoking**, as the risk of recurrence is 50% in patients who smoke. High altitudes, flying in unpressurized aircraft, and scuba diving should also be avoided. Thoracoscopy or open thoracotomy with stapling or laser pleurodesis is indicated with recurrent spontaneous pneumothorax, any bilateral pneumothorax, or failure of tube thoracostomy. Scarification by abrasion of the pleural surface may produce pleural symphysis.

Complications   Approximately 30% of patients with spontaneous pneumothorax develop recurrent episodes regardless of initial therapy (observation versus tube thoracostomy). Recurrence is uncommon following surgical interventions. Spontaneous pneumothorax may be complicated by **pneumomediastinum or subcutaneous emphysema**; a secondary ruptured esophagus or bronchus should be ruled out. Tension pneumothorax may rarely be complicated by acute respiratory failure, cardiopulmonary arrest, or death.

ID/CC	A **40-year-old African-American female** complains of progressive **dyspnea on exertion, cough, chest discomfort, weight loss**, and loss of appetite.
HPI	The patient also complains of a purplish rash over her face. Her symptoms have progressed over the past year. She is a **nonsmoker**.
PE	VS: low-grade fever (38.2°C); tachypnea. PE: mild **respiratory distress; bluish-purple, swollen lesions** on nose, cheeks, and earlobes (LUPUS PERNIO); clubbing; bilateral fine inspiratory crackles.
Labs	CBC: lymphopenia. ESR elevated; **hypercalcemia**; hyperglobulinemia; serum **ACE levels elevated**. UA: 24-hour urine calcium elevated. Skin and transbronchial lung biopsies reveal **noncaseating granulomas**; staining and cultures negative for organisms. PFTs: reduced DL_{co}; reduced FEV_1 and FVC; FEV_1/FVC ratio normal (**restrictive pattern of disease**); **Kveim–Siltzbach test** (antigen from human sarcoid tissue injected intradermally) positive.
Imaging	**[A]** CXR: **bilateral hilar lymphadenopathy**. **[B]** Later stage of lymphadenopathy (1) and reticulonodular densities. HRCT: presence of lymphadenopathy and pulmonary fibrosis confirmed. Nuc: gallium-67 lung scan positive (demonstrates diffuse uptake).
Pathogenesis	The etiology of sarcoidosis is unknown. Accumulation of T cells, macrophages, and noncaseating granulomas in affected organs are seen, probably secondary to an exaggerated immune response to self-antigens or persistent foreign antigens. Organs most commonly affected are the **lungs, skin, eye, and lymph nodes**.

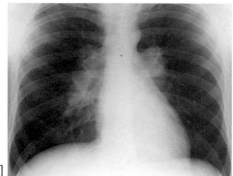

[A]

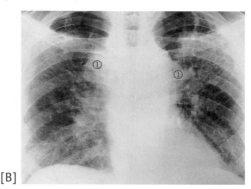

[B]

SARCOIDOSIS

Epidemiology   Sarcoidosis occurs worldwide but is 10 times more prevalent and severe among **African Americans** than among whites. Individuals 20 to 40 years old are most often affected, with a slightly higher prevalence found among females. It is more common in **temperate climates** than in tropical zones and has a higher incidence among **nonsmokers**.

Management   Most patients are asymptomatic or undergo spontaneous remission within 2 years. Use **corticosteroids** for symptomatic pulmonary involvement, systemic symptoms, hypercalcemia, or involvement of extrapulmonary tissues that leads to organ dysfunction, iritis, and CNS and cardiac involvement. **Immunosuppressants** (e.g., methotrexate, azathioprine) may be effective. Regular clinical evaluation is required.

Complications   Neurologic (peripheral neuropathy, cranial nerve palsies, papilledema, meningitis, epilepsy, cerebellar ataxia), cardiac (arrhythmias, CHF, cardiomyopathy), and ocular (anterior or posterior uveitis) manifestations may occur. Hypopituitarism, arthritis, cor pulmonale, and nephrocalcinosis occur as well.

Atlas Link   U C V 1   PM-P2-092

MINICASE 215: PULMONARY EOSINOPHILIA SYNDROMES

Pneumonia characterized by eosinophilic infiltrates
- can be idiopathic or secondary to parasitic infections (e.g., *Strongyloides*, toxocariasis), drug reactions (e.g., penicillin, sulfa drugs), *Aspergillus* infections, Churg–Strauss vasculitis, or asthma
- presents with dyspnea, fever, sputum production, and wheezing
- serum eosinophilia
- CXR reveals pulmonary infiltrates, atelectasis secondary to mucous plugs, and possibly bronchiectasis in chronic disease
- treat with corticosteroids for severe symptoms, bronchodilators for asthma exacerbation, antibiotics for fungal or parasitic infection

ID/CC	A 52-year-old man presents with increasing **shortness of breath on exertion**.
HPI	The patient's medical history includes no cardiac or pulmonary disease. He has been working in the **stone-cutting** industry for more than 25 years. His dyspnea on exertion has progressed over many years, and he denies any smoking, alcohol use, or illicit drug use. His family history is unremarkable.
PE	VS: normal. PE: well developed and in no acute distress; no JVD, carotid bruits, or lymphadenopathy; **fine inspiratory crackles at the bases of lungs bilaterally**; cardiac exam normal with no extra heart sounds or murmurs; extremities notable only for **digital clubbing**; no cyanosis or edema.
Labs	PFTs: mild obstructive and restrictive disease and decreased DL_{co}.
Imaging	CXR: diffuse ground-glass, nodular infiltrates with small, rounded opacities (silicotic nodules) throughout the lung; **peripheral calcifications in hilar lymph nodes** ("EGGSHELL CALCIFICATIONS") may be noted. CT, chest: multiple small nodules.
Pathogenesis	Silicosis represents a diffuse fibrotic reaction of the lungs to inhalation of free crystalline silica particles that are ingested by alveolar macrophages, which rupture and subsequently release cytotoxic enzymes. The silica is reingested by other macrophages, continuing a cycle of cytotoxic enzyme release and progressive local fibrotic reactions, ultimately producing acellular fibrous nodules characteristic of the clinical disease. Long-term exposure over 15 to 20 years results in fibrosis that is sufficient to produce characteristic small, rounded opacities in the upper lobes with retraction, hilar adenopathy, and "eggshell calcifications."
Epidemiology	Exposure to free silica or crystalline quartz occurs through major occupational hazards such as rock mining, stone cutting, foundry work, quarrying (especially granite), tunneling, sandblasting, pottery making, and packing of silica flour. Progressive pulmonary fibrosis occurs in a dose-response fashion after many years. However, individuals working in small spaces can develop silicosis following periods of exposure as limited as 10 months.
Management	Cessation of silica exposure often necessitates a change in occupation. **Corticosteroids** may improve the chronic lymphocytic alveolitis. Screen for tuberculosis with tuberculin

SILICOSIS

skin test and CXR, as patients with silicosis are clearly at **greater risk of acquiring** *Mycobacterium tuberculosis* (silicotuberculosis) as well as atypical mycobacterial infections. Multidrug treatment is indicated for any patient with a positive tuberculin test or old, healed tuberculous scars on CXR.

Complications Progressive fibrosis may lead to coalescence of large irregular masses exceeding 1 cm in diameter (progressive massive fibrosis), leading to significant functional impairment with severe **restrictive and obstructive disease** on pulmonary function testing. Respiratory failure may follow within a few years. Atypical silicates such as talc may cause **pleural or lung cancers**.

Atlas Links ⬜CⓋ🔲 PM-P2-093, PG-P2-093

MINICASE 216: α_1-ANTITRYPSIN DEFICIENCY

Variable deficiency of enzyme that inhibits trypsin, elastase, and collagenase, causing proteolytic destruction of lung and liver in variable combinations
- presents with panacinar emphysema or hepatic cirrhosis
- PFTs reveal $FEV_1/FVC < 75\%$
- liver biopsy shows cirrhosis
- treat emphysema with home oxygen, human α_1-trypsin replacement therapy may be indicated in some patients
- only transplant can treat liver disease

ID/CC A **21-year-old male** complains of **low back pain** and **stiffness**.

HPI He states that the pain is associated with **morning stiffness** that gradually **improves with exercise**. He also complains of **fatigue, weight loss**, and hip and shoulder pain.

PE VS: low-grade fever. PE: pallor; **stooped posture**; reduced inspiratory chest excursion; high-pitched, blowing **diastolic murmur** (aortic insufficiency); prominent abdomen; fixed kyphosis; **poor lumbar spinal mobility; loss of lumbar lordosis; sacroiliac joint tenderness**.

Labs CBC: anemia (Hct 30%). Low serum iron and TIBC (anemia of chronic disease); elevated ESR and C-reactive protein; elevated IgA; **negative rheumatoid factor and ANA**; positive **HLA-B27**.

Imaging **[A]** XR: **periarticular sclerosis** with blurred sacroiliac joint margins. **[B]** XR, spine: ankylosis and fusion of spinal vertebral bodies (BAMBOO SPINE) and sacroiliac joints.

Pathogenesis Ankylosing spondylitis (AS) is characterized by the presence of **inflammatory arthritis** of the **axial skeleton** (classically **sacroiliitis**) that may be accompanied by **peripheral arthritis, enthesitis**

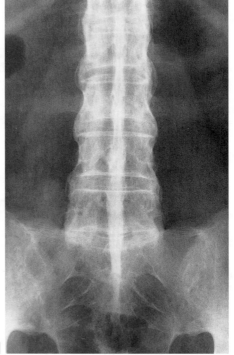

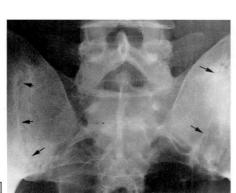

[A]   [B]

(inflammation at the site of tendinous or ligamentous attachment to bone), recurrent acute anterior **uveitis, aortic valve incompetence**, or pulmonary fibrosis. The precise etiology is unknown, but **immune-mediated mechanisms** are likely given the close association with HLA-B27, elevated serum levels of IgA and acute phase reactants, and an inflammatory histology. There is a significant association of AS with inflammatory bowel disease.

Epidemiology   AS usually begins in the second to third decade, is three times more common in **males** than in females, and is more prevalent among first-degree relatives who inherit the B27 allele.

Management   **NSAIDs** (indomethacin and, in those who fail to respond, phenylbutazone) are the first line of therapy. Patients must **eliminate cigarette smoking**, initiate a **physical therapy** and **exercise** regimen, receive **genetic counseling**, and minimize spinal trauma to prevent fractures. Immunosuppressants and corticosteroids are of limited or no utility.

Complications   Complications include **spinal fractures and spondylodiscitis** after minimal trauma, and **hip and knee deterioration** necessitating hip or knee replacement. Patients with long-standing disease may develop **aortic insufficiency, conduction defects**, deteriorating vision secondary to recurrent **uveitis** (40% of cases), pulmonary fibrosis, or chronic prostatitis.

MINICASE 217: BAKER'S CYST

Cyst arising from the synovial lining of the knee
- commonly associated with rheumatoid arthritis
- presents with painful swelling of the popliteal fossa, often mimicking thrombophlebitis
- treat with NSAIDs and leg elevation, consider triamcinolone injection

---

MINICASE 218: BEHÇET'S DISEASE

An idiopathic autoinflammatory disease affecting young adults
- presents with recurrent aphthous ulcers, genital ulcers, and anterior uveitis as well as with rashes and large joint arthritis
- treat with systemic glucocorticoids
- complications include blindness

ID/CC   A **45-year-old female** complains of chronic progressive **muscle weakness** and **tenderness** associated with a diffuse **rash**.

HPI   She is now unable to get up from a sitting position and also has **difficulty raising her arms and climbing stairs** (proximal muscle weakness). She also complains of difficulty swallowing (DYSPHAGIA).

PE   PE: diffuse erythema over the face, neck, shoulders and upper chest/back (SHAWL SIGN) and maculopapular eruptions; scaly patches over dorsum of PIP and metacarpal joints (GOTTRON'S SIGN); **lilac-colored** rash on eyelids (HELIOTROPE) with periorbital edema; decreased strength in proximal muscle groups.

Labs   Markedly **elevated CK; elevated aldolase**; elevated ESR. UA: myoglobinuria. EMG: low amplitude, short duration motor unit action potentials. Muscle biopsy shows **inflammation** and muscle fiber **necrosis**.

Imaging   XR, soft tissues: diffuse soft tissue calcifications.

Pathogenesis   Dermatomyositis is characterized by the presence of **polymyositis** in association with characteristic **skin changes**. Profound proximal muscle weakness, dysphagia, **respiratory impairment**, and **myocarditis** are key characteristics. The precise etiology is unknown, although viral infection, genetic factors, and autoimmunity are thought to be contributory mechanisms. Polymyositis/dermatomyositis may occur in **association with neoplasia** (breast, gynecologic, or rectal), vasculitis, or other connective tissue diseases (usually progressive systemic sclerosis, rheumatoid arthritis, mixed connective tissue disease, and SLE).

Epidemiology   May develop at any age, with a peak incidence between the fifth and sixth decades of life; **females outnumber males** by a ratio of 2 to 1. The 5-year survival rate is approximately 75%. Poor prognostic factors include delayed treatment, severe disease at initial presentation, underlying malignancy, associated connective tissue diseases, and the presence of antibodies to Jo-1 and signal recognition peptide.

Management   **Corticosteroids** are first-line agents; with improvement beginning as early as 1 to 4 weeks following the initiation of treatment. Measure progress with **serum enzymes. Cytotoxic drugs** (cyclophosphamide, methotrexate, and cyclosporine) may be

DERMATOMYOSITIS

used in refractory disease. Strength exercises and physical therapy are critical once control of the disease process is established.

Complications Death may result from cardiac, pulmonary, or renal complications. Patients may have persistent muscle weakness, atrophy, or contracture.

Atlas Links ⓤⒸⓋ2 IM2-051A, IM2-051B

MINICASE 219: DECOMPRESSION SICKNESS

Results from the effects of gas (predominantly nitrogen) bubbles on tissues and cells formed by a rapid reduction in pressure while ascending at the end of a dive
- clinical presentation is divided into three categories: type 1 (mild), type 2 (severe), and arterial gas embolization
- may present with joint pain (bends), pruritus, and a sharply defined area of pallor on the tongue (Liebermeister sign), or may progress to pulmonary symptoms, hypovolemic shock, nervous system involvement, and even death
- treat with 100% oxygen, recompression therapy, hyperbaric oxygen, and hydration
- complications include residual paralysis, myocardial necrosis, and other ischemic injuries

---

MINICASE 220: DRUG-INDUCED LUPUS

A reversible lupus-like syndrome most often caused by procainamide, hydralazine, isoniazid, methyldopa, and quinidine
- presents with malar rash, arthralgias, and pericardial friction rub
- anti-histone antibody positive
- kidneys and CNS are usually spared
- treat by removing the offending agent
- steroids may be used for severe symptoms
- the disease is self-limiting

MINICASE 221: FELTY'S SYNDROME

Systemic rheumatoid arthritis coupled with splenomegaly and neutropenia
- presents with infections, purpura, and splenomegaly
- neutropenia and thrombocytopenia
- abdominal CT demonstrates enlarged spleen
- treat the underlying rheumatoid arthritis, splenectomy may ameliorate disease

ID/CC   A **45-year-old male** presents to the clinic complaining of **severe pain in the right big toe**.

HPI   He states that he has had similar attacks in the past, each of which came on suddenly.

PE   VS: low-grade fever (38.3°C). PE: **tophi** in helix of ear and in hands and feet; **olecranon bursitis** bilaterally; **exquisitely tender, erythematous, swollen, shiny, and warm right first MTP joint** (PODAGRA).

Labs   Serum **uric acid elevated**; synovial fluid aspiration reveals **negatively birefringent crystals** and elevated WBC (20,000).

Imaging   XR, foot: **punched-out erosions of bone** and **overhanging edge of new bone** at the MTP joint of the big toe. XR, hand: soft tissue swelling (due to tophus) of the PIP joint of the index finger.

Pathogenesis   Gout is characterized by the presence of hyperuricemia with resultant **arthritis** (usually monoarticular/inflammatory and presenting as repetitive acute episodes), **tophaceous deposition** in peri- and intra-articular locations, **urate nephropathy** (due to urate crystal deposition in interstitial renal parenchyma), and **nephrolithiasis.** Hyperuricemia may result from **increased dietary intake** of purines in foods such as liver and kidney; **increased de novo synthesis** of purines due to increased activity of PRPP synthetase enzyme; increased breakdown of purines into uric acid due to a **deficiency of HGPRT**-mediated nucleotide salvage mechanism, as in Lesch–Nyhan syndrome; **accelerated purine nucleotide degradation** associated with conditions of rapid cell turnover (tumor lysis syndrome, myeloproliferative diseases, hemolysis, or rhabdomyolysis); or **undersecretion** (most individuals with gout have **defective uric acid clearance**). In acute gout, elevated uric acid levels lead to the development of microtophi, which are shed into the joint space and are subsequently coated by immunoglobulins and complement, promoting phagocytosis by neutrophils. The crystals disrupt the phagosomal membranes, causing lysosomal enzyme release into the joint space and enhancing inflammation.

Epidemiology   Gout arises primarily in **middle-aged and elderly men, postmenopausal women**, and patients with **end-stage renal disease**. Gout is seen more frequently with obesity, diabetes mellitus, hypertension, type II and type IV hyperlipidemia, and atherosclerosis.

Additionally, gout may be precipitated by surgery, illness, or excessive alcohol consumption.

Management	**Colchicine, NSAIDs**, or **intra-articular glucocorticoids** for acute attacks; **allopurinol prophylaxis and uricosuric drugs (probenecid)** for chronic hyperuricemia. Encourage patients to avoid alcohol (inhibits urate excretion) and foods high in purines (e.g., shellfish).
Complications	Nephrolithiasis, renal impairment, destructive arthropathy, and GI bleeding (secondary to high-dose NSAIDs).
Atlas Links	UCV2 IM2-052A, IM2-052B UCV1 PM-BC-094

MINICASE 222: MIXED CONNECTIVE TISSUE DISORDER

An idiopathic syndrome with variable characteristics of SLE, systemic sclerosis, polymyositis, and rheumatoid arthritis
- presents with Raynaud's phenomenon, arthritis, skin disease, and diffuse organ disease
- anti-U1RNP antibodies
- treat with corticosteroids, NSAIDs

MINICASE 223: OSTEOPOROSIS

Quantitative reduction of total skeletal bone mass due to increased bone resorption
- usually seen in postmenopausal women (preventable with postmenopausal estrogen replacement)
- commonly presents with spinal compression fractures, wrist fractures, hip fractures, or acquired kyphosis
- DEXA scan reveals diminished bone density
- x-rays of the spine may reveal kyphosis and osteoporotic collapse of mid- to lower thoracic and lumbar vertebrae
- treat with calcium supplements, estrogen, bisphosphonates, and exercise
- complications include fractures, loss of height, kyphosis

Atlas Link: UCV1 PG-P3-085

ID/CC	A **52-year-old male** complains of **weight loss, malaise**, fatigue, headache, and **muscle pain** of 6 months' duration.
HPI	He has no significant past medical history.
PE	VS: **fever** (38.5°C); hypertension (BP 178/95). PE: mild pallor; **diffuse palpable purpura**.
Labs	CBC: anemia (Hct 33%); leukocytosis (13,000); **thrombocytosis**; no eosinophilia. Elevated ESR; hypergammaglobulinemia; **positive hepatitis B surface antigen**. UA: mild **proteinuria**; hematuria; **cellular casts**. Biopsy shows **necrotizing inflammation of small and medium-size arteries**.
Imaging	**[A]** Angio, abdominal: **multiple aneurysms of small and medium-size blood vessels**.
Pathogenesis	Polyarteritis nodosa is characterized by **necrotizing inflammation of small and medium-sized** arteries (such as renal and visceral arteries). **PMN infiltrates** are prevalent in the **acute stage** of the

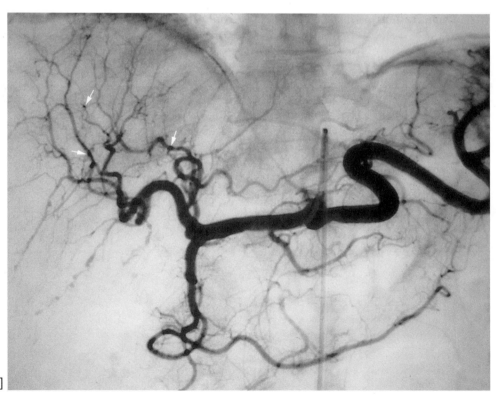

[A]

POLYARTERITIS NODOSA

disease, whereas **mononuclear infiltrates** mark the **chronic stage** of illness. Fibrinoid necrosis later compromises the lumen, causing aneurysmal dilatation, thrombosis, and subsequent infarction of the tissues. Clinical manifestations indicate the organ system involvement: glomerular arteriolitis may present as hypertension and azotemia; vasa nervorum (arteries supplying nerves) involvement may present as mononeuritis multiplex; and cardiac involvement may present as MI or CHF. The frequent presence of hepatitis B surface antigen suggests an immunologic component.

Epidemiology   A relatively uncommon illness that **presents between the fourth and fifth decades** with a male-to-female ratio of approximately 2 to 1. Associations have been found with SLE, rheumatoid arthritis, hepatitis B virus infection, hairy cell leukemia, and serous otitis media.

Management   **Prednisone** in combination with **cyclophosphamide** has been shown to be effective. Early initiation of treatment is key. The **control of hypertension** is critical for reducing the morbidity and mortality of cardiac, renal, and CNS complications.

Complications   Death usually results from renal failure, GI complications (bowel infarct), and cardiovascular manifestations. Untreated polyarteritis nodosa has a 100% mortality rate.

MINICASE 224: POLYMYALGIA RHEUMATICA

An inflammatory condition whose median age of onset is 70
- female-to-male ratio is 2:1
- associated with HLA-DR4 and giant cell (temporal) arteritis
- presents with aches in the shoulder, hip girdle muscles, and proximal extremities that worsen in the morning
- elevated ESR and normochromic anemia
- treat with corticosteroids

ID/CC A **36-year-old male** complains of **swelling and pain** in the right **knee** and left **ankle** for the past 2 weeks.

HPI He reports having suffered a severe case of *Salmonella* **enterocolitis** approximately 1 month ago. He also has **burning on urination** (due to urethritis), irritated eyes, occasional fever, and **moderate weight loss**.

PE VS: **fever** (38.6°C). PE: mild clear, watery **conjunctival discharge;** mild **stomatitis**; tenderness to palpation, swelling, and erythema in right knee and left ankle with slight effusion.

Labs CBC/Lytes: normal. **ESR moderately elevated; RA factor negative**; synovial fluid culture negative; positive **HLA-B27**.

Imaging XR: permanent or progressive joint disease in peripheral joints (articular soft tissue swelling, joint space narrowing, marginal erosions) and in sacroiliac joints.

Pathogenesis Reiter's syndrome is characterized by the presence of **asymmetric "reactive arthritis"** (affecting large weight-bearing joints such as the knees and ankles or **sacroiliitis), conjunctivitis** or **uveitis, urethritis** (commonly a nongonococcal venereal infection), and **mucocutaneous lesions** (such as balanitis, stomatitis, and keratoderma blennorrhagicum). The presence of **HLA-B27** and characteristic x-ray findings are highly suggestive of the diagnosis of Reiter's syndrome.

Epidemiology Affects men and women equally following a dysenteric infection (*Salmonella, Shigella, Yersinia, Campylobacter*) or primarily males following an STD (*Chlamydia trachomatis* or *Ureaplasma urealyticum*) within the previous months. Classified as a form of reactive arthritis.

Management **NSAIDs** for symptomatic relief. Use **corticosteroids** as needed. It is not known if antibiotics are effective in preventing this syndrome; however, it has been shown that prompt antibiotic administration for chlamydial urethritis may be beneficial. **Tetracycline** used for 3 months may reduce symptom duration and is particularly useful owing to its combination of antimicrobial and anti-inflammatory effects. **Sulfasalazine** is used for patients who are unresponsive to NSAIDs and antibiotic regimens.

REITER'S SYNDROME

Complications   Complications include urethral strictures, permanent joint damage, cataracts, carditis, aortic regurgitation, and **aortic root dissection**. Relapse is common.

MINICASE 225: POLYMYOSITIS

Inflammation of skeletal muscle
- 10% of cases are associated with coexisting malignancy
- presents with progressive proximal muscle weakness with atrophy and associated skin findings in dermatomyositis (heliotrope rash, Gottron's papules, photosensitive skin rash)
- elevated CPK
- EMG and muscle biopsy (showing myonecrosis and perivascular mononuclear infiltrates) are suggestive
- treat with high-dose corticosteroids, methotrexate, seek the underlying malignancy

---

MINICASE 226: PROGRESSIVE SYSTEMIC SCLEROSIS (SCLERODERMA)

An idiopathic autoimmune fibrosing disorder
- presents with diffuse skin fibrosis with telangiectasis, Raynaud's phenomenon, dysphagia, and cardiac and renal problems
- treat with corticosteroids for acute exacerbations
- penicillamine may be helpful

Atlas Links: UCV2 **MC-226**   UCV1 PM-P3-089, PG-P3-089

MINICASE 227: PSORIATIC ARTHRITIS

Autoimmune arthritis seen in patients with psoriasis
- presents with asymmetric large and small joint arthritis
- commonly affects the DIP joints of the fingers
- waxing and waning course
- patients are often HLA-B27 positive
- treat the underlying skin disease, NSAIDs for arthritis
- complications include severe joint erosions

ID/CC A **45-year-old woman** complains of **vague pain and stiffness** in her **wrists** and **hands** for the past several years.

HPI Her pain is most **prominent in the morning**, with stiffness typically lasting for more than 1 hour. She reports that her symptoms have progressed, as manifested by the formation of "bumps" (RHEUMATOID NODULES) on her **fingers, wrists**, and **elbows**. She additionally notes increased malaise, weight loss, and generalized weakness.

PE VS: normal. PE: extremities with decreased range of motion and swelling around **bilateral PIP and MCP joints**; flexion of DIP with extension of PIP (SWAN-NECK DEFORMITY); mild effusion and tenderness in both ankles; **[A]** ulnar deviation of digits at MCP joints with relative sparing of DIP joints; subcutaneous nodules over bony prominences; hyperextension of DIP with flexion of PIP (BOUTONNIERE DEFORMITY); subcutaneous nodules on both elbows.

Labs CBC: normocytic, normochromic anemia; slight elevation in WBC and platelet counts. ESR moderately elevated; positive **rheumatoid factor**; elevated C-reactive protein; joint fluid with moderate elevation in WBC count (5,000 to 50,000/μL) and > 50% PMNs on differential; negative culture.

Imaging **[B]** XR, hand: **periarticular osteoporosis** with **erosions** around the affected MCP and PIP joints. **[C]** Another case, more advanced, demonstrates arthritis mutilans, including ulnar deviation of the fingers and carpal fusion.

Pathogenesis Rheumatoid arthritis (RA) is a chronic inflammatory disorder of **autoimmune** origin that is characterized by **synovitis of multiple joints** with **pannus formation**. Granulation tissue eventually erodes the cartilage, bone, ligaments, and tendons; scarring, contracture, and deformity result from inflammatory destruction of these structures. Any joint may be involved, but the **PIP, MCP, wrists, knees, ankles, and toes** are most commonly affected.

Epidemiology Rheumatoid arthritis is a common disease that **affects females three times more often than males**. The age of onset is usually 20 to 40 years, with prevalence increasing with age, although RA may present at any age. A strong association with **HLA-DR4** has been observed.

Management **Aspirins/NSAIDs** are first-line therapy unless contraindicated. If these treatment modalities are unsuccessful, **immunosuppressive agents** such as methotrexate, gold salts, hydroxychloroquine, sulfasalazine or azathioprine may be tried. Oral corticosteroids should be reserved for unresponsive cases, extra-articular disease or to relieve symptoms while waiting for the effect of immunosuppressive agents. Intra-articular corticosteroids may be tried when only one or two joints are inflamed. Key **nonpharmacologic measures** include weight loss, education, exercise, and assistive devices.

Complications Complications include **atlantoaxial dislocation**, pleuropulmonary disease **(pleural effusion, pulmonary nodules, Caplan's syndrome)**, pericarditis, **Felty's syndrome** (RA associated with splenomegaly and neutropenia), **vasculitis,** and pharmacologic therapy-related side effects (e.g., aspirin/**NSAID-induced GI hemorrhage**). Factors associated with premature death include long length of disease, prolonged steroid use, early age at diagnosis, and low socioeconomic status.

Atlas Link 󠀀UCV2󠀀 IM2-055

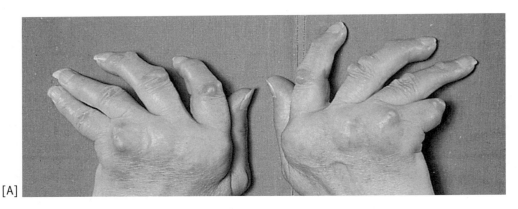

[A]

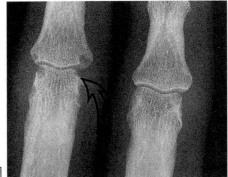

[B]

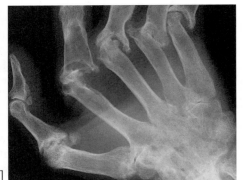

[C]

ID/CC	A **34-year-old female** presents to her physician with a **butterfly-shaped rash** over the bridge of her nose and cheeks that is **made worse by sunlight** (PHOTOSENSITIVITY).
HPI	The patient states that she has been experiencing increasing **malaise, fatigue, shortness of breath**, muscle aches, **joint pain**, swelling, and early-morning stiffness over the past 2 months.
PE	VS: fever (38.9°C). PE: diffuse **maculopapular rash** over arms, back, and chest; raised, erythematous **malar rash** over cheeks and nose, extending to ears; **painless oral ulcers**; movements of knees, wrists, and joints of the hands are restricted and painful.
Labs	CBC: normocytic, normochromic anemia; leukopenia. **ANA positive; elevated ESR; anti-Sm** and **anti-dsDNA antibodies** detected; serum C2, C4 complement factors decreased. UA: proteinuria; hematuria; cellular casts (due to lupus **nephritis**).
Imaging	CXR: small right **pleural effusion**. Echo: no signs of pericarditis or pericardial effusion.
Pathogenesis	Systemic lupus erythematosus (SLE) is a disease of unknown etiology in which cells and tissues are damaged by **immune complexes** and **autoantibodies**. Lack of suppression by typical immunoregulatory systems produces **abnormal hyperactivity** of T and B cells. It is thought that genetic susceptibility, sex hormones, and exogenous antigens influence abnormal self-tolerance in these patients and promote immune cell activation. The antigens that stimulate autoantibodies are both **endogenous** and **exogenous**. Criteria for the diagnosis of SLE include **any four** of the following manifestations: malar rash, discoid rash, photosensitivity, oral ulcers, arthritis, serositis, ANAs, or renal, neurologic, hematologic, and immunologic disorders. The diagnosis of SLE can only be made after drug-induced lupus syndrome has been ruled out.
Epidemiology	Ninety percent of patients with SLE are **women**, typically of **childbearing years**. However, men, children, and the elderly can be affected. Prevalence is higher among **African Americans**. Sex hormones are thought to influence immune tolerance.
Management	Complete remission of SLE is rare. Patients with arthritis, mild pleurisy, and mild pericarditis should be treated with **NSAIDs** only. Use **antimalarial** drugs (retinal damage should be monitored) or **low-dose corticosteroids** for skin and musculoskeletal

SYSTEMIC LUPUS ERYTHEMATOSUS (SLE)

involvement. Life-threatening or severe SLE should be treated with **high-dose corticosteroids; cytotoxic agents** such as azathioprine, chlorambucil, and cyclophosphamide are useful for suppression of active disease and lowering the quantity of steroids needed. End-stage glomerulonephritis and clotting disorders may not respond to drug therapy.

Complications   Complications include **vasculitic lesions**, including purpura, ulcers, urticaria, and gangrene of the digits; **lupus nephritis**; cognitive dysfunction and seizures with **CNS complications**; ARDS and intra-alveolar hemorrhage; and pancreatitis, abdominal discomfort, diarrhea, vasculitis, and peritonitis. Pericarditis, myocarditis, effusions, arrhythmias, and infarction are manifestations of **cardiac lupus; pleural effusions** may lead to atelectasis, pneumonitis, and infection.

Atlas Links   `UCV2` IM2-056   `UCV1` PM-P3-095

MINICASE 228: SJÖGREN'S SYNDROME

Autoimmune destruction of exocrine glands, often associated with other autoimmune disease (e.g., rheumatoid arthritis, SLE, scleroderma)
- primarily affects middle-aged women
- presents with dry mouth and eyes, parotid enlargement, and denuded corneal epithelium
- hypergammaglobulinemia
- ANA and RF positive
- treatment is supportive (e.g., eye drops)

MINICASE 229: TAKAYASU'S ARTERITIS

Medium- and large-vessel arteritis
- common in young Asian females
- presents with fatigue, fever, and decreased peripheral pulses
- increased ESR and elevated immunoglobulin levels
- arteriography demonstrates inflammatory aneurysms
- treat with corticosteroids

SYSTEMIC LUPUS ERYTHEMATOSUS (SLE)

ID/CC   A **42-year-old** Caucasian female presents with increasing **sinus pain, bloody nasal discharge**, and **difficulty breathing**.

HPI   The patient adds that she has been experiencing **hemoptysis, shortness of breath**, and general chest discomfort. She also complains of increasing malaise, weakness, loss of appetite, and weight loss. One month ago she started having pain in her left ear with gradual hearing loss and bloody discharge (**otitis media**) that did not respond to a 10-day course of antibiotics.

PE   VS: low-grade fever (38.1°C); tachypnea (RR 24). PE: episcleritis; nasal mucosa ulcerated with bloody discharge; coarse breath sounds bilaterally.

Labs   CBC: leukocytosis and mild anemia. **ESR markedly elevated; antineutrophil cytoplasmic antibodies** (ANCAs; C-ANCA more specific) present; biopsy of lung lesion reveals necrotizing granulomatous vasculitis. UA: **proteinuria** and **hematuria** (secondary to **glomerulonephritis**).

Imaging   CXR: cavitating nodules.

Pathogenesis   Wegener's granulomatosis (WG) is characterized by **granulomatous vasculitis** of the **upper and lower respiratory tracts** with **glomerulonephritis**. Lung involvement appears as multiple, nodular cavitary infiltrates. Upper airway lesions, especially in the sinuses, demonstrate necrosis, inflammation, and granuloma formation.

Epidemiology   WG is a rare disease that affects men and women equally. The disease rarely affects patients before adolescence; mean age of onset is 40 years.

Management   The treatment of choice is **cyclophosphamide** given in combination with **steroids**. WBC count and renal function should be closely monitored. Remissions can be induced in most patients; long-term follow-up is required.

Complications   Focal and segmental glomerulitis may progress into a **rapidly progressive crescentic glomerulonephritis**; nasal ulceration may produce **septal perforation** that may result in **saddle-nose deformity**. Eye complications can produce episcleritis, scleritis, and sclerouveitis.

Atlas Link   [U][C][V][1] PM-P3-096

WEGENER'S GRANULOMATOSIS

MINICASE 230: TEMPOROMANDIBULAR JOINT SYNDROME

Believed to be a stress-related disorder caused by grinding of the teeth (BRUXISM), resulting in muscle spasm and pain
- presents with pain and tenderness in the muscles of mastication and in the TMJ as well as with crepitus when the joint is moved, decreased range of motion, headaches, and earaches
- treat with NSAIDs or benzodiazepines
- complications include alterations in dentition, chronic facial pain, and malocclusion

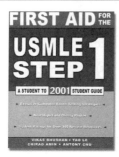
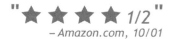
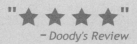
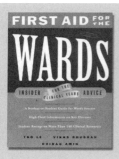
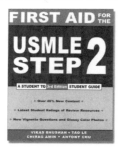
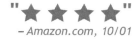
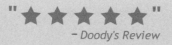
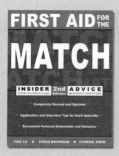